PLANT BASED FOODS TO FUEL THE CANCER FIGHT

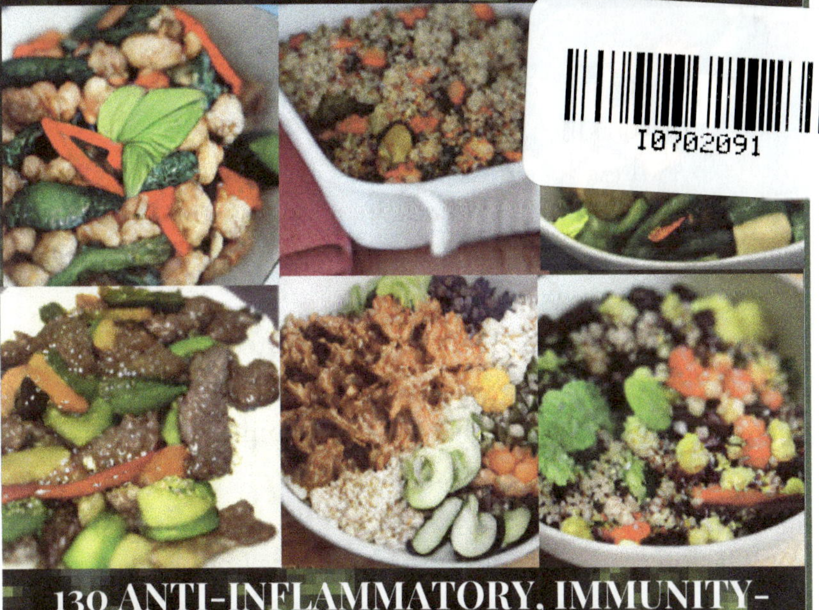

130 ANTI-INFLAMMATORY, IMMUNITY-BOOSTING RECIPES PACKED WITH ORGANIC FRUITS, VEGETABLES, LEGUMES, AND PHYTONUTRIENTS

ADELINE GREEN

Copyright © 2024 by Adeline Green

Disclaimer

Table of Contents

Introduction

In the tapestry of life, health is the most precious thread, weaving through our moments, our dreams, and our aspirations. As we navigate the complexities of our modern world, the resonance of good health becomes ever more pronounced, and for many, the formidable specter of cancer stands as one of the greatest challenges to that harmony.

In this journey toward optimal well-being, "Plant-Based Foods to Fuel the Cancer Fight" emerges as a beacon of hope and empowerment. Imagine a culinary odyssey where every meal is a deliberate act of self-love, a step toward bolstering our bodies in the face of adversity. This book is more than a collection of recipes; it is a guide to a transformative way of life, intricately designed to harness the healing power of nature.

The Challenge: A Battle Against Cancer

Cancer, with its silent intrusion into our lives, often leaves us feeling powerless. Yet, within this challenge lies the potential for resilience, strength, and healing. "Plant-Based Foods to Fuel the Cancer Fight" addresses the pressing need for a proactive approach to health, intertwining the profound connection between nutrition and our body's ability to defend itself.

The Solution: 130 Anti-Inflammatory, Immunity-Boosting Recipes

Embark on a journey where food becomes your ally in the fight against cancer.

This book presents not merely a collection of recipes but a symphony of flavors meticulously composed to combat inflammation, boost immunity, and nurture your body at its core. With 130 recipes crafted from organic fruits, vegetables, legumes, and phytonutrient-rich ingredients, each page is a step toward reclaiming control over your health.

Benefits of the Book: Empowering You on Your Health Odyssey

Transformative Recipes: Unleash the power of nature's bounty with recipes designed to not only tantalize your taste buds but also fortify your body against the challenges of cancer.

Educational Insights: Navigate the intricate relationship between diet and cancer with accessible insights, empowering you to make informed choices for a healthier life.

Holistic Wellness: Beyond the kitchen, discover a holistic approach to wellness, addressing the emotional and psychological facets of the cancer journey.

As you turn the pages of "Plant-Based Foods to Fuel the Cancer Fight," envision not just a book but a lifeline, connecting you to a world where each meal is a celebration of life, resilience, and the unwavering spirit to conquer adversity. Let this be your invitation to a journey where the simple act of eating becomes a profound act of self-love and healing. Welcome to a new chapter in your health odyssey – let the journey begin.

Chapter 1
Understanding Cancer and Nutrition

The Connection Between Diet and Cancer

In the intricate dance of life, the relationship between diet and cancer emerges as a profound and complex duet. This chapter is a voyage into the realms where the choices we make at the dining table resonate in the cellular symphony of our bodies. Join me as we unravel the threads connecting nutrition and the intricate landscape of cancer.

Embarking on the Journey: From Cells to Cuisine

Imagine our bodies as vibrant ecosystems, each cell a player in the intricate harmony of health. Now, picture the nutrients from the food we consume as the notes that compose this symphony. The connection between diet and cancer lies in the subtle interplay of these notes, influencing the cellular narrative in ways both subtle and profound.

Understanding the Cellular Dialogue: At a microscopic level, the cells in our bodies engage in a constant dialogue. This communication extends beyond mere survival; it orchestrates the delicate balance between health and disease. The food we consume, laden with nutrients and antioxidants, contributes to this dialogue, influencing the cellular script in ways that can either promote or hinder the growth of cancer cells.

In this exploration, antioxidants and phytonutrients emerge as the unsung heroes in our culinary journey. These compounds, generously bestowed by nature upon fruits, vegetables, and whole grains, act as defenders, shielding our cells from the oxidative stress that can fuel the growth of cancer. Picture them as guardians, standing resilient against the tempest of cellular imbalance.

The Culinary Canvas: The palette of a cancer-fighting diet is vibrant, boasting a rich spectrum of colors, textures, and flavors. From the deep greens of kale to the ruby reds of berries, each ingredient is a stroke on the culinary canvas, contributing to a masterpiece of nourishment and protection.

Bridging Science and Sensibility
As we navigate the scientific undercurrents, let's not lose sight of the human aspect. Understanding the connection between diet and cancer is not just about parsing data; it's about empowering ourselves with informed choices. It's a call to recognize the agency we hold in shaping our well-being through the meals we craft.

Empowerment through Knowledge: Knowledge becomes our ally, empowering us to make conscious decisions that extend beyond the realms of taste and satisfaction. It's a realization that our dietary choices are not just about fueling the body but about fostering an environment where health can flourish, and cancer finds resistance.

Phytonutrients and Their Impact on Cellular Health

In the enchanting world of plant-based nutrition, phytonutrients stand as nature's gift to our cells, weaving a tale of resilience, defense, and vibrant health. As we embark on this exploration, let's peel back the layers of understanding to reveal the profound impact of these bioactive compounds on the intricate dance of cellular health.

The Essence of Phytonutrients:

Derived from the Greek word "phyto," meaning plant, phytonutrients are the bioactive compounds that plants produce to defend themselves against environmental stressors. Remarkably, these compounds extend their protective embrace to us when we incorporate plant-based foods into our diets.

A Symphony of Colors and Flavors:

Picture a rainbow on your plate, a kaleidoscope of colors emanating from fruits, vegetables, nuts, and seeds. Each hue signifies a unique phytonutrient profile, and collectively, they compose a symphony of flavors that not only tantalize our taste buds but also fortify our cellular defenses.

The Cellular Ballet:

Within the microscopic theater of our cells, phytonutrients perform a delicate ballet. They act as antioxidants, neutralizing free radicals that can otherwise wreak havoc on cellular structures.

By mitigating oxidative stress, phytonutrients help to maintain the integrity of our cellular machinery, fostering an environment where health can thrive.

Categories of Phytonutrients and Their Roles:
1. Flavonoids: Abundant in fruits, vegetables, and teas, flavonoids exhibit antioxidant and anti-inflammatory properties, contributing to heart health and overall well-being.

2. Carotenoids: Think of the vibrant orange in carrots and the deep green in spinach. Carotenoids, such as beta-carotene, lutein, and zeaxanthin, not only lend color but also support eye health and immune function.

3. Glucosinolates: Predominantly found in cruciferous vegetables like broccoli and kale, glucosinolates have been associated with cancer prevention, particularly in supporting detoxification pathways.

4. Polyphenols: Gracing foods like berries, dark chocolate, and green tea, polyphenols showcase antioxidant prowess, promoting heart health and aiding in the fight against chronic diseases.

Unlocking the Healing Potential:
Phytonutrients are not merely passive spectators; they actively participate in our wellness journey. Their impact transcends the confines of conventional nutrition, reaching into the realms of preventive medicine and holistic health.

Incorporating Phytonutrients into Your Diet:

The journey toward optimal cellular health begins at your plate. Embrace a diverse array of colorful, whole foods. Experiment with herbs and spices. Savor the nuanced flavors that signify the presence of these botanical guardians.

As we dive into the essence of phytonutrients, let's celebrate the kaleidoscope of flavors, colors, and health benefits that they bring to our tables. This chapter is an invitation to not only understand but to actively integrate these plant-powered compounds into our daily lives, cultivating a symphony of cellular health that resonates through every aspect of our well-being.

Organic Foods and Their Benefits in Cancer Prevention

In the pursuit of a nourishing and health-conscious lifestyle, the choice to embrace organic foods emerges as a conscious step towards wellness. This chapter unravels the intricate tapestry of organic foods and illuminates the tangible benefits they offer in the realm of cancer prevention.

The Essence of Organic:

Organic foods, cultivated through methods that eschew synthetic pesticides, fertilizers, and genetically modified organisms (GMOs), represent a commitment to purity and sustainability. Beyond a mere label, the organic journey is a celebration of harmonious coexistence with nature.

Guardians of Cellular Integrity:

In the orchestra of cancer prevention, organic foods play a crucial role as guardians of cellular integrity. By steering clear of synthetic pesticides and harmful chemicals, these foods minimize the risk of exposure to potential carcinogens, creating a protective shield around our cells.

The Benefits Unveiled:

1. Reduced Chemical Exposure: Organic farming practices prioritize natural alternatives to chemical pesticides and fertilizers. This reduction in chemical exposure is especially significant, considering the potential links between certain agricultural chemicals and cancer risk.

2. Enhanced Nutrient Density: Organic foods often boast higher nutrient levels, offering a more concentrated source of vitamins, minerals, and antioxidants. These nutritional powerhouses contribute to overall health and bolster the body's defense mechanisms.

3. Supporting a Balanced Microbiome: The health of our gut microbiome is intricately linked to our overall well-being. Organic foods, free from synthetic additives, may promote a healthier balance of beneficial bacteria in the digestive system, fostering an environment less conducive to inflammation, a key player in cancer development.

4. Antioxidant Richness: Organic fruits and vegetables have been shown to contain higher levels of certain antioxidants. These compounds act as warriors against oxidative stress, a process implicated in the initiation and progression of cancer.

Navigating the Organic Landscape:

Embracing a Whole-Food Approach: The heart of an organic lifestyle lies not just in the absence of synthetic inputs but also in a holistic embrace of whole, unprocessed foods. This journey involves savoring the richness of seasonal produce, exploring local markets,.

Decoding Labels: Understanding organic certifications and labels empowers you to make informed choices. Look for trusted seals such as USDA Organic or equivalent certifications in your region, ensuring that your choices align with the standards of organic agriculture.

A Call to Conscious Consumption:

In exploring the benefits of organic foods in cancer prevention, this chapter extends an invitation—to not only fill our plates but also to cultivate a mindful relationship with the food we consume. As we embrace the organic narrative, let it be a testament to the belief that our daily choices, both on and off the plate, have the power to shape a future where wellness and cancer prevention walk hand in hand.

Chapter 2
Getting Started with Plant-Based Eating

Transitioning to a Plant-Based Diet

In the symphony of dietary choices, transitioning to a plant-based diet is akin to tuning into the harmonious rhythm of nature. This chapter serves as a guide for those embarking on the transformative journey of embracing plant-powered living. Let's unravel the threads of transition, weaving a narrative that nurtures not just the body but also the spirit.

The Plant-Based Palette: A Vibrant Tapestry of Choices

Begin with Exploration: Transitioning to a plant-based diet is not a rigid leap but rather a journey of exploration. Start by acquainting yourself with the kaleidoscope of plant-based foods, vibrant fruits, crisp vegetables, wholesome grains, and legumes that dance on your plate. Embrace the diversity that nature offers, allowing your palate to awaken to new textures and flavors.

Gradual Shifts: Transitioning need not be an abrupt departure from your existing dietary habits. Consider introducing plant-based meals gradually. Perhaps start with one plant-based day a week or designate certain meals as plant-focused. This gradual approach allows your taste buds and digestive system to acclimate, making the transition a more enjoyable and sustainable experience.

Building Your Plant-Powered Pantry: Foundations for Success
Stocking Essentials: A well-prepared pantry is your ally in the plant-based adventure. Fill your shelves with whole grains like quinoa and brown rice, an array of colorful lentils and beans, nuts, seeds, and an abundance of herbs and spices. These staples form the foundation of nourishing plant-based meals and open up a world of culinary possibilities.

Flavorful Substitutes: Explore plant-based substitutes for animal products. Experiment with tofu, tempeh, and seitan as protein alternatives. Dive into the world of nut-based cheeses and milk alternatives. These flavorful substitutes not only enhance your culinary repertoire but also provide the nutrients essential for a balanced plant-based diet.

Navigating Challenges: Empathy in Your Transition
Understanding the Journey: Transitioning to a plant-based diet can present challenges, both practical and emotional. Recognize that the journey is unique for each individual. Approach yourself with empathy and understanding, acknowledging that changes take time. Celebrate the progress, no matter how small, and embrace the learning curve with a sense of curiosity.

Addressing Nutritional Concerns: Ensure a balanced transition by paying attention to essential nutrients. While plant-based diets offer a wealth of nutrients, it's essential to plan for sufficient intake of protein, vitamin B12, iron, and omega-3 fatty acids.

Consider consulting a nutrition professional to tailor your plant-based journey to your unique nutritional needs.

Creating a Plant-Based Lifestyle: Beyond the Plate

Holistic Living: Plant-based eating extends beyond the plate, it's a lifestyle that embraces holistic well-being. Engage in mindful practices such as yoga, meditation, and mindful eating. Foster a connection with the environment by exploring local farmers' markets and embracing sustainable living practices. As you transition, let it be not just a change in diet but a celebration of a vibrant and conscious way of life.

In the realm of transitioning to a plant-based diet, this chapter is your compass, a guide that illuminates the path, acknowledges the challenges, and invites you to savor the joys of discovering a plant-powered way of living. Embrace the journey, one plant-based meal at a time, as you embark on a transformative adventure that harmonizes with the wisdom of nature and the well-being of your body and soul.

Stocking Your Kitchen with Essential Ingredients

In the heart of your home lies a realm of possibilities, a space where the alchemy of plant-based cooking comes to life. Stocking your kitchen with essential ingredients is the first step in crafting a vibrant and nourishing plant-based culinary journey. Let's open the doors to your plant-powered pantry and discover the essentials that will transform your kitchen into a haven of health and creativity.

Foundations of a Plant-Based Pantry:

Whole Grains: Begin with the wholesome embrace of whole grains. Quinoa, brown rice, farro, and oats are versatile foundations that form the backbone of plant-based meals. Rich in fiber and nutrients, these grains provide sustained energy and a satisfying base for a variety of dishes.

Lentils and Legumes: Elevate your protein game with an assortment of lentils, chickpeas, black beans, and red kidney beans. Packed with protein, fiber, and essential minerals, legumes add substance and heartiness to your meals, ensuring a well-rounded plant-based diet.

Nuts and Seeds: Enrich your pantry with the crunch and nutrition of nuts and seeds. Almonds, walnuts, chia seeds, flaxseeds, and sunflower seeds offer a spectrum of flavors and essential fatty acids. Incorporate them into salads, smoothies, or as finishing touches for various dishes.

Flavors that Dance: Herbs and Spices

Herbs: Fresh herbs infuse your meals with bursts of flavor and vibrant color. Keep staples like basil, cilantro, parsley, and mint on hand. These aromatic wonders add freshness to salads, soups, and entrees, elevating the sensory experience of your plant-based creations.

Spices: Dive into the enchanting world of spices—cumin, coriander, turmeric, paprika, and cinnamon. These culinary treasures not only awaken your taste buds but also contribute diverse health benefits. Experiment with spice blends to create depth and complexity in your dishes.

Plant-Powered Proteins and Substitutes:

Tofu and Tempeh: Embrace the versatility of tofu and tempeh as protein-rich alternatives. These soy-based wonders absorb the flavors of your marinades and lend themselves to an array of savory and sweet dishes. Grilled, baked, or sautéed, they become the canvas for your culinary creativity.

Plant-Based Dairy Alternatives: Explore the wide array of plant-based milk alternatives—almond, soy, oat, coconut, and cashew. These dairy substitutes seamlessly integrate into recipes, providing a creamy texture and an abundance of nutrients. Nutritional yeast is another gem to add a cheesy flavor to your plant-based creations.

The Fresh Bounty: Fruits and Vegetables

Seasonal Produce: Embrace the vibrant colors and textures of seasonal fruits and vegetables. From leafy greens and cruciferous vegetables to juicy berries and citrus delights, the freshness of produce forms the heart of your plant-based kitchen. Aim to include a variety of colors to ensure a diverse range of nutrients.

Root Vegetables: Potatoes, sweet potatoes, carrots, and beets add substance and natural sweetness to your meals. Roasted, mashed, or spiralized, these root vegetables offer a comforting and hearty foundation for plant-based dishes.

Pantry Staples for Convenience:

Canned Tomatoes: Keep a stock of canned tomatoes for quick and easy sauces, stews, and soups. Tomatoes are a versatile ingredient that imparts depth and umami to your plant-based creations.

Whole-Grain Pasta and Rice Noodles: For convenient yet wholesome meal options, whole-grain pasta and rice noodles are invaluable. Pair them with a medley of vegetables and a flavorful sauce for a satisfying plant-based feast.

Your Plant-Powered Toolkit: Kitchen Equipment

High-Speed Blender: A blender becomes your ally in creating creamy smoothies, sauces, and soups. Invest in a high-speed blender for a seamless blending experience.

Food Processor: A food processor simplifies the process of chopping, slicing, and dicing, saving you time in meal preparation. From nut butter to veggie burgers, the food processor is a versatile companion.

Navigating Your Plant-Based Culinary Adventure:
As you stock your kitchen with these essential ingredients, envision it as a canvas waiting to be painted with vibrant hues of plant-based goodness. Let creativity be your guide, and embrace the joy of exploring new flavors, textures, and culinary horizons. In the realm of plant-based cooking, your kitchen is not just a space for nourishment but a sanctuary where the art of healthy living and gastronomic delight converges.

Planning Balanced Plant-Based Meals

In the culinary adventure of plant-based eating, the art of planning balanced meals takes center stage. This chapter is a compass, guiding you through the harmonious orchestration of nutrients, flavors, and textures. Let's embark on a journey where every plate is a canvas, and each meal is a celebration of plant-powered nourishment.

The Symphony of Nutrient Balance: Crafting a Plant-Based Plate

Embracing the Rainbow: Picture your plate as a canvas, and the array of colors from fruits and vegetables as the palette. Aim to include a spectrum of colors, each hue representing a unique set of phytonutrients, vitamins, and minerals. The diversity in colors ensures a broad range of nutrients, promoting overall health and vitality.

Plant-Powered Proteins: Elevate your meals with plant-based proteins. Legumes, lentils, chickpeas, tofu, and tempeh are stellar sources of protein, offering essential amino acids crucial for muscle health and overall well-being. Diversify your protein intake for optimal nutritional balance.

The Wholesome Harmony: Carbohydrates and Whole Grains

Whole Grains: Integrate whole grains into your meals for sustained energy and a hearty foundation. Quinoa, brown rice, farro, and whole-grain pasta are versatile options that complement the flavor profile of plant-based dishes. These grains contribute fiber, aiding in digestion and promoting a feeling of fullness.

Abundant Vegetables: Let vegetables shine as the focal point of your meals. Whether roasted, sautéed, or enjoyed raw, vegetables provide essential vitamins, minerals, and fiber. They add texture, flavor, and a nutritional boost to your plant-based creations.

Fats that Nourish: Healthy Plant-Based Oils

Plant-Based Oils: Choose heart-healthy plant-based oils such as olive oil, avocado oil, and coconut oil to add richness and beneficial fats to your meals. These oils provide essential fatty acids and enhance the absorption of fat-soluble vitamins present in plant foods.

Nuts and Seeds: Sprinkle a handful of nuts and seeds onto your dishes for both texture and nutrition. Almonds, walnuts, chia seeds, and flaxseeds are excellent sources of omega 3 fatty acids, promoting brain health and overall well-being.

Flavorful Accents: Herbs, Spices, and Condiments

Herbs and Spices: Elevate the taste profile of your plant-based meals with an array of herbs and spices. Cumin, coriander, turmeric, basil, and mint bring depth and complexity to your dishes. Experiment with spice blends to discover flavor combinations that delight your palate.

Condiments: Explore plant-based condiments to add zing to your meals. Tahini, balsamic vinegar, soy sauce, and nutritional yeast are flavorful additions that enhance the taste of salads, sauces, and dressings without compromising on health.

Meal Planning Strategies for Success:

Batch Cooking: Streamline your plant-based journey with batch cooking. Prepare grains, legumes, and roasted vegetables in larger quantities and store them for convenient use throughout the week. This time-saving strategy ensures that wholesome, plant-based ingredients are readily available.

Balanced Plate Approach: Adopt the balanced plate approach by visually dividing your plate into sections. Reserve one-half for colorful vegetables, one-quarter for whole grains, and one-quarter for plant-based proteins. This method promotes a harmonious distribution of nutrients and flavors.

Savoring the Journey: Mindful Eating Practices

Mindful Eating: Beyond the nutritional aspect, embrace the practice of mindful eating. Engage your senses, savor each bite, and be present in the culinary experience. Mindful eating fosters a deeper connection with your food, promotes better digestion, and encourages a healthier relationship with nourishment.

Navigating Your Plant-Based Culinary Odyssey:

As you plan and savor balanced plant-based meals, remember that the journey is as important as the destination. Embrace the creativity, relish the flavors, and celebrate the nourishment that plant-based eating brings to your life. Let each meal be a testament to the art of crafting balanced, plant-powered plates that not only nourish the body but also delight the soul.

Chapter 3
Breakfast Delights
Energizing Smoothie Bowls
Recipe 1. Tropical Paradise Bliss Bowl

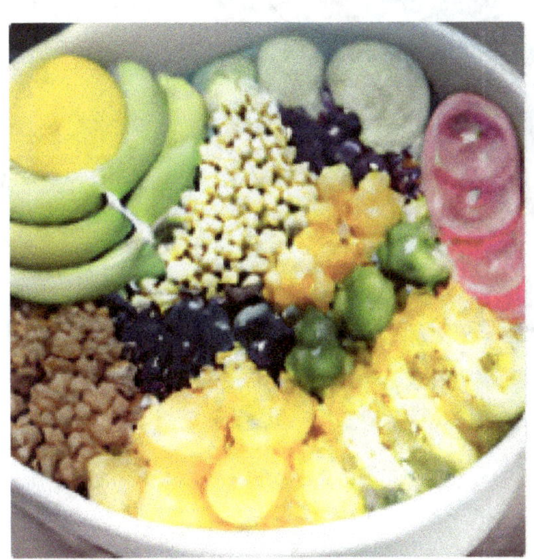

Ingredients:

- 1 cup frozen mango chunks
- 1/2 cup frozen pineapple chunks
- 1 banana
- 1/2 cup coconut water

Preparation:

1. Blend mango, pineapple, banana, and coconut water until smooth.
2. Pour into a bowl and adorn with kiwi slices, shredded coconut, and a sprinkle of chia seeds.

Toppings:

Kiwi slices, shredded coconut, chia seeds

Recipe 2. Berry Burst Power Bowl

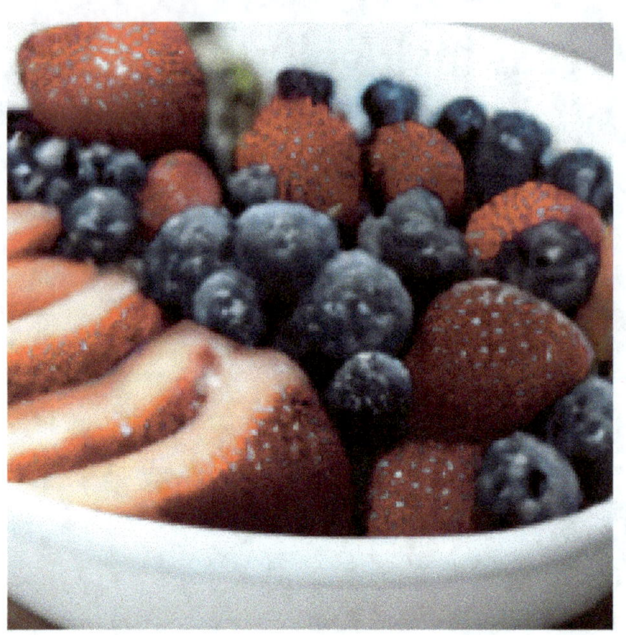

Ingredients:

- 1 cup mixed berries (strawberries, blueberries, raspberries)
- 1/2 cup almond milk
- 1 tablespoon almond butter
- 1 tablespoon chia seeds

Toppings:

Granola, sliced almonds, fresh berries

Preparation:

1. Blend mixed berries, almond milk, almond butter, and chia seeds until creamy.
2. Gently transfer to a serving bowl and garnish with a generous sprinkle of granola, toasted almond slivers, and a vibrant medley of fresh berries.

Recipe 3. Green Goddess Smoothie Bowl

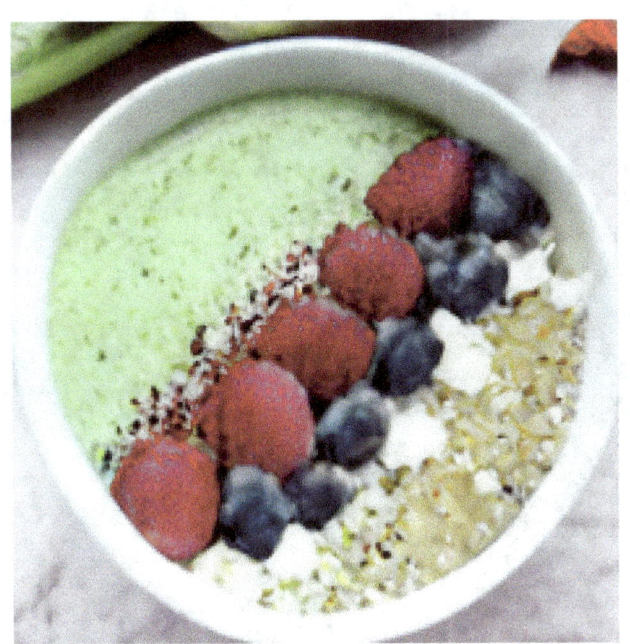

Ingredients:

- 1 cup spinach leaves
- 1/2 avocado
- 1/2 cup green grapes
- 1/2 cup coconut water

Preparation:

1. Blend spinach, avocado, green grapes, and coconut water until silky.
2. Transfer to a bowl and garnish with sliced kiwi, hemp seeds, and sliced almonds.

Toppings:

Sliced kiwi, hemp seeds, sliced almonds

Recipe 4. Chocolate Banana Bliss Bowl

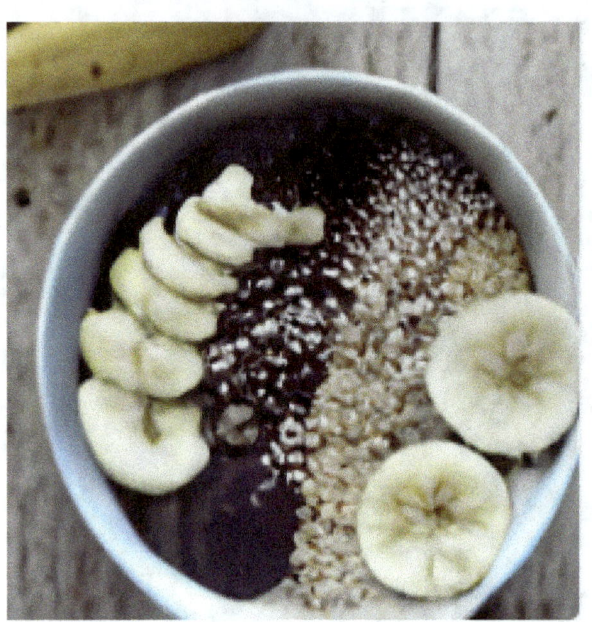

Ingredients:

- 2 ripe bananas
- 2 tablespoons cacao powder
- 1/2 cup almond milk
- 1 tablespoon peanut butter

Preparation:

1. Blend ripe bananas, cacao powder, almond milk, and peanut butter until velvety.
2. Pour into a bowl and top with cocoa nibs, banana slices, and chopped nuts.

Toppings:

Cocoa nibs, banana slices, chopped nuts

Recipe 5. Citrus Sunrise Smoothie Bowl

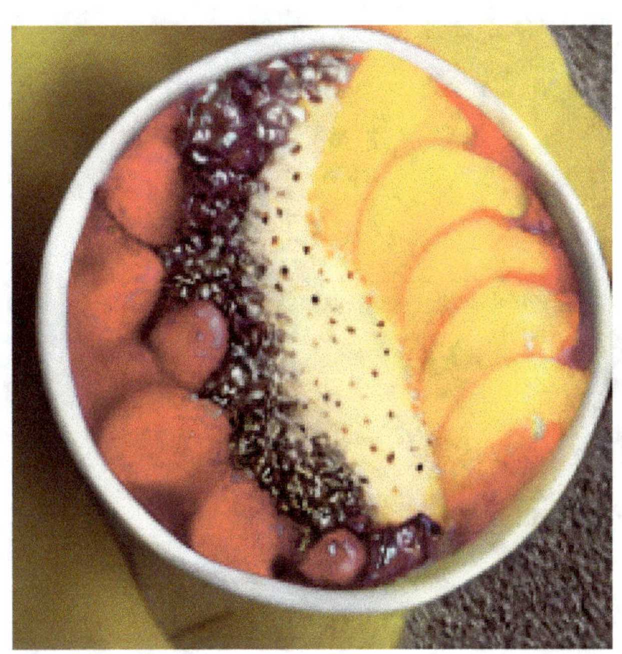

Ingredients:

- 1 cup orange segments
- 1/2 cup mango chunks
- 1/2 cup Greek yogurt (or plant-based yogurt)
- 1 tablespoon honey

Preparation:

1. Blend orange segments, mango chunks, Greek yogurt, and honey until smooth.
2. Transfer to a bowl and decorate with citrus slices, granola, and a sprinkle of bee pollen.

Toppings:

Citrus slices, granola, bee pollen

Recipe 6. Peanut Butter Banana Crunch Bowl

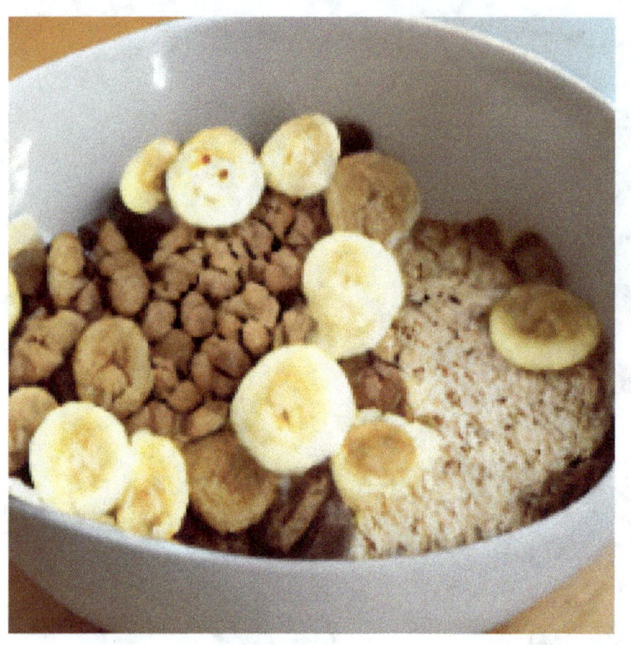

Ingredients:

- 2 frozen bananas
- 2 tablespoons peanut butter
- 1/2 cup almond milk
- 1 tablespoon flaxseeds

Preparation:

1. Blend frozen bananas, peanut butter, almond milk, and flaxseeds until creamy.
2. Spoon into a bowl and garnish with sliced bananas, granola, and chopped peanuts.

Toppings:

Sliced bananas, granola, chopped peanuts

Recipe 7. Acai Berry Bliss Bowl

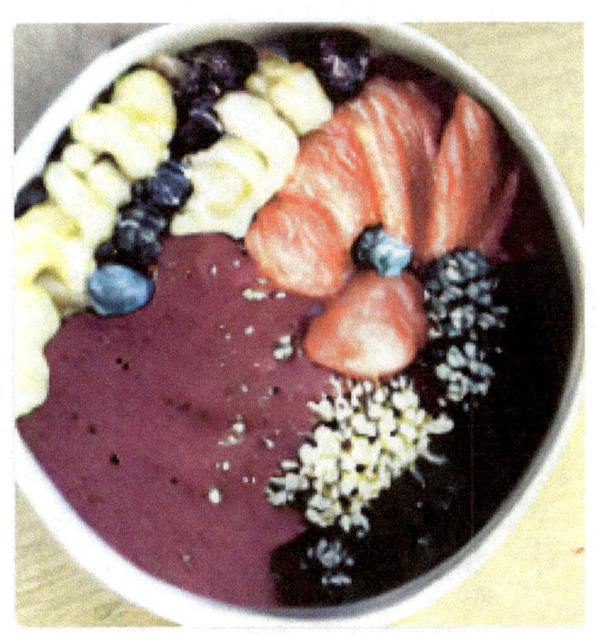

Ingredients:

- 1 packet frozen acai puree
- 1/2 cup mixed berries
- 1/2 cup coconut water
- 1 tablespoon almond butter

Preparation:

1. Blend acai puree, mixed berries, coconut water, and almond butter until smooth.
2. Pour into a bowl and top with sliced strawberries, coconut flakes, and pumpkin seeds.

Toppings:

Sliced strawberries, coconut flakes, pumpkin seeds

Recipe 8. Peachy Keen Delight Bowl

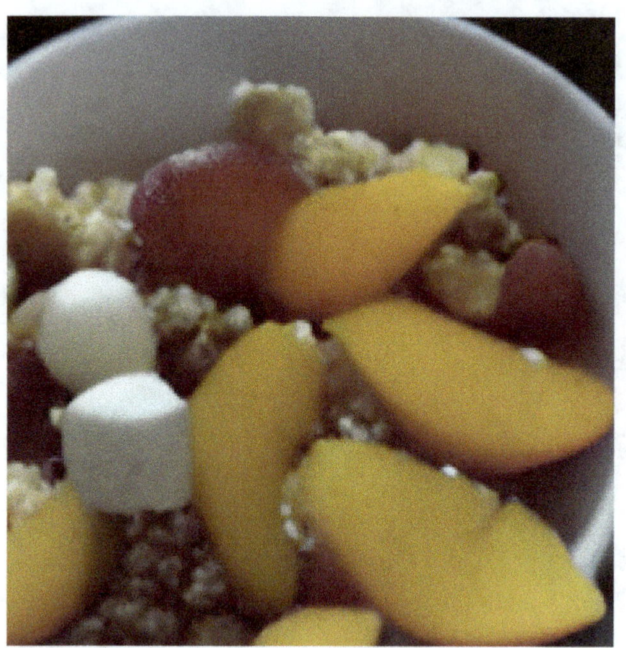

Ingredients:

- 1 cup frozen peaches
- 1/2 cup mango chunks
- 1/2 cup orange juice
- 1 tablespoon chia seeds

Preparation:

1. Blend frozen peaches, mango chunks, orange juice, and chia seeds until luscious.
2. Transfer to a bowl and adorn with fresh peach slices, granola, and sliced almonds.

Toppings:

Fresh peach slices, granola, sliced almonds

Recipe 9. Blueberry Banana Bonanza Bowl

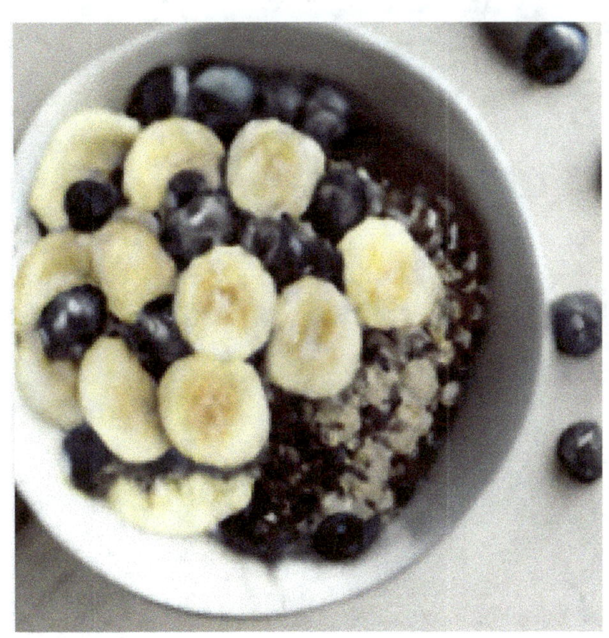

Ingredients:

- 1 cup blueberries
- 1 banana
- 1/2 cup almond milk
- 1 tablespoon almond butter

Preparation:

1. Blend blueberries, banana, almond milk, and almond butter until velvety.
2. Spoon into a bowl and embellish with blueberry compote, hemp seeds, and crushed pistachios.

Toppings:

Blueberry compote, hemp seeds, crushed pistachios

Recipe 10. Mocha Madness Smoothie Bowl

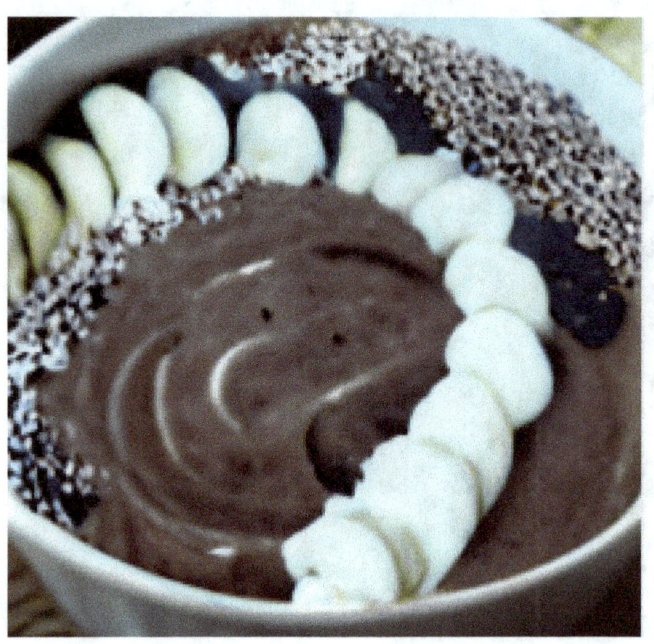

Ingredients:

- 1 cup cold brew coffee
- 2 tablespoons cacao powder
- 1 frozen banana
- 1/2 cup plant-based milk

Preparation:

1. Blend cold brew coffee, cacao powder, frozen banana, and plant-based milk until decadent.

2. Transfer to a bowl and crown with espresso beans, cacao nibs, and a dollop of coconut whipped cream.

Toppings:

Espresso beans, cacao nibs, coconut whipped cream

Wholesome Oatmeal Variations

Recipe 1. Classic Maple Cinnamon Oats

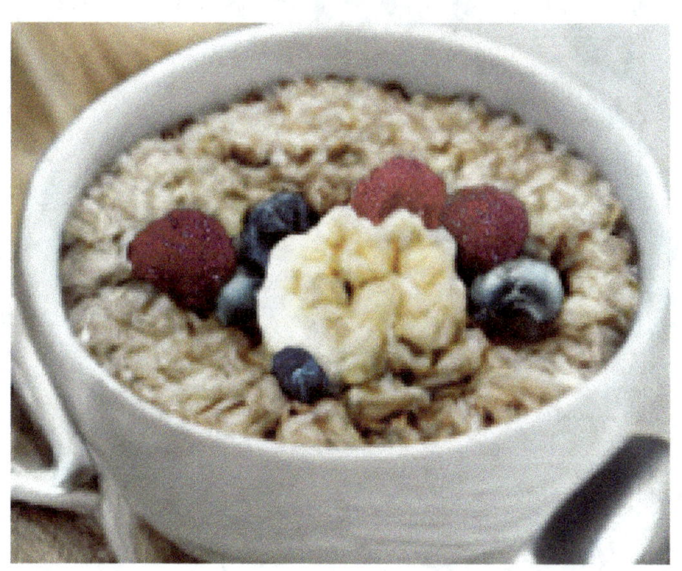

Ingredients:

- 1/2 cup rolled oats
- 1 cup almond milk
- 1 tablespoon pure maple syrup
- 1/2 teaspoon ground cinnamon

Preparation:

1. Combine rolled oats, almond milk, maple syrup, and cinnamon in a saucepan.
2. Cook over medium heat until creamy. Top with sliced bananas, chopped nuts, and an extra drizzle of maple syrup.

Toppings:

Sliced bananas, chopped nuts, a drizzle of additional maple syrup

Recipe 2. Apple Pie Oatmeal Delight

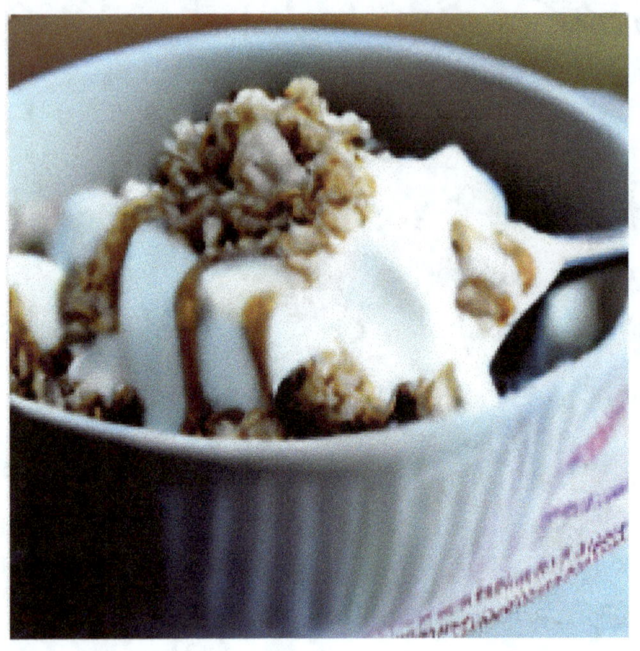

Ingredients:

- 1/2 cup old-fashioned oats
- 1 cup apple juice
- 1/2 apple, diced
- 1/2 teaspoon ground cinnamon

Preparation:

1. Cook old-fashioned oats in apple juice, adding diced apples and ground cinnamon.
2. Simmer until the oats are tender. Garnish with additional diced apples, a sprinkle of cinnamon, and a handful of granola.

Toppings:

Diced apples, a sprinkle of cinnamon, granola

Recipe 3. Berry Bliss Overnight Oats

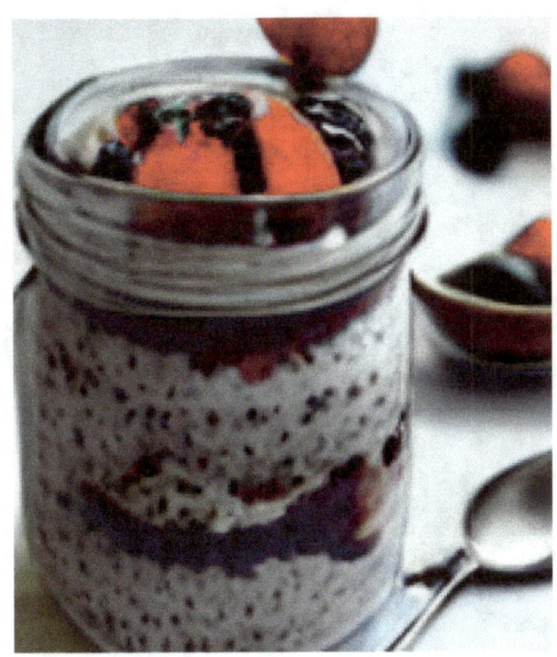

Ingredients:

- 1/2 cup rolled oats
- 1/2 cup almond milk
- 1/2 cup mixed berries (strawberries, blueberries, raspberries)
- 1 tablespoon chia seeds

Preparation:

1. Mix rolled oats, almond milk, mixed berries, and chia seeds in a jar.
2. Refrigerate overnight. In the morning, layer with fresh berries, a dollop of yogurt, and a drizzle of honey.

Toppings:

Fresh berries, a dollop of yogurt, honey

Recipe 4. Peanut Butter Banana Crunch Oats

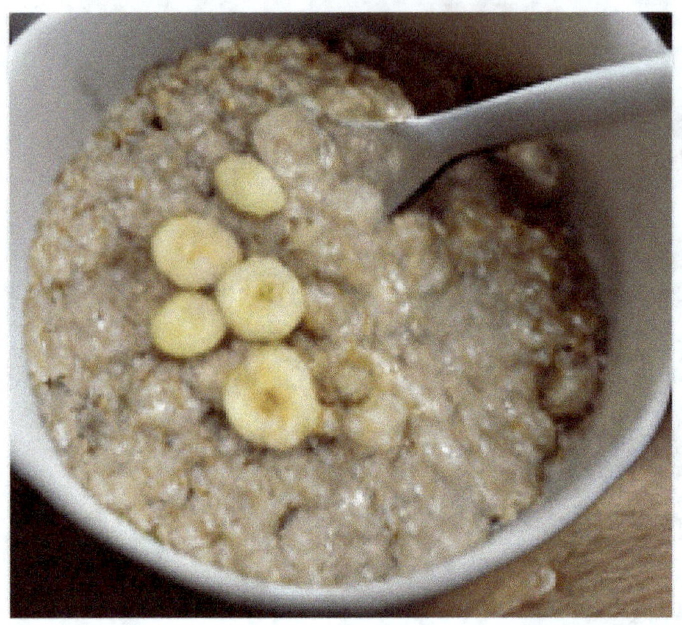

Ingredients:

- 1/2 cup steel-cut oats
- 1 cup water
- 1 banana, mashed
- 1 tablespoon peanut butter

Preparation:

1. Cook steel-cut oats in water, incorporating mashed banana and peanut butter.
2. Stir until creamy. Top with sliced bananas, chopped peanuts, and a swirl of peanut butter.

Toppings:

Sliced bananas, chopped peanuts, a swirl of peanut butter

Recipe 5. Coconut Almond Joy Oatmeal

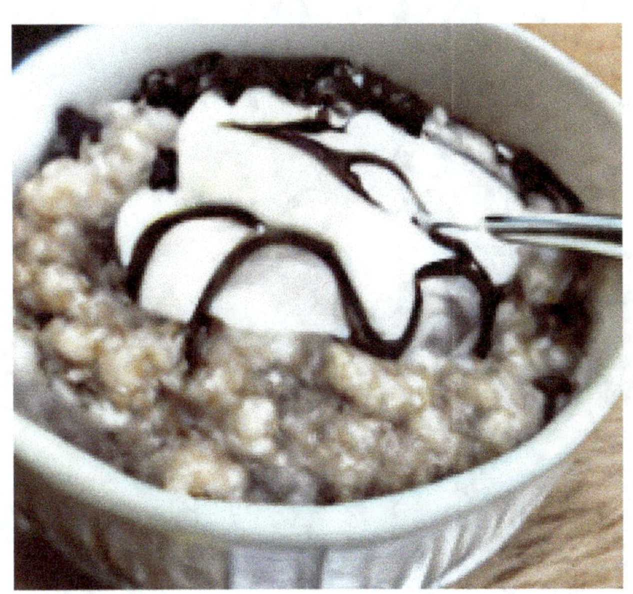

Ingredients:

- 1/2 cup old-fashioned oats
- 1 cup coconut milk
- 1 tablespoon cocoa powder
- 1 tablespoon almond butter

Toppings:

Shredded coconut, sliced almonds, chocolate shavings

Preparation:

1. Combine old-fashioned oats, coconut milk, cocoa powder, and almond butter.
2. Simmer, stirring occasionally, until the oats reach a texture you enjoy.
3. Garnish with shredded coconut, sliced almonds, and chocolate shavings.

Recipe 6. Savory Mushroom and Spinach Oats

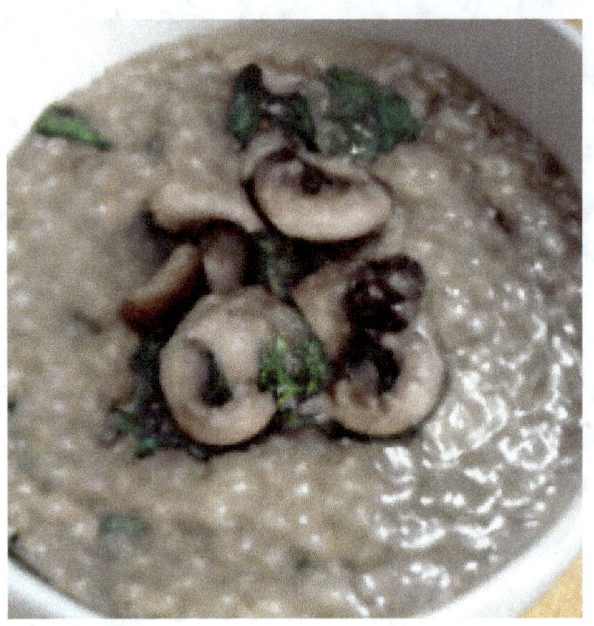

Ingredients:

- 1/2 cup rolled oats
- 1 cup vegetable broth
- 1/2 cup sautéed mushrooms
- Handful of fresh spinach

Toppings:

Sliced cherry tomatoes, a sprinkle of nutritional yeast, fresh herbs

Preparation:

1. Cook rolled oats in vegetable broth, folding in sautéed mushrooms and fresh spinach. Simmer until the oats are tender.
2. Top with sliced cherry tomatoes, a sprinkle of nutritional yeast, and fresh herbs.

Recipe 7. Pumpkin Spice Latte Oatmeal

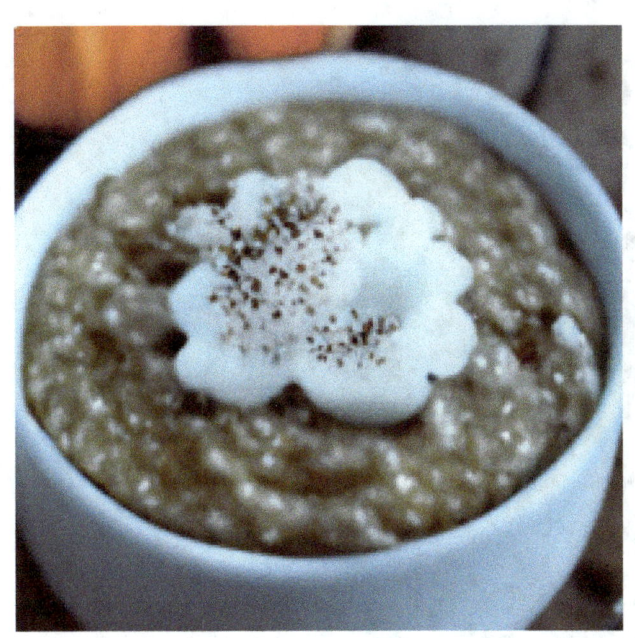

Ingredients:

- 1/2 cup steel-cut oats
- 1 cup brewed coffee
- 2 tablespoons pumpkin puree
- 1/2 teaspoon pumpkin spice

Preparation:

1. Cook steel-cut oats in brewed coffee, blending in pumpkin puree and pumpkin spice. Stir until creamy.
2. Finish with pepitas, a swirl of coconut cream, and a sprinkle of cinnamon.

Toppings:

Pepitas, a swirl of coconut cream, a sprinkle of cinnamon

Recipe 8. Mediterranean-inspired olive and Tomato Oats

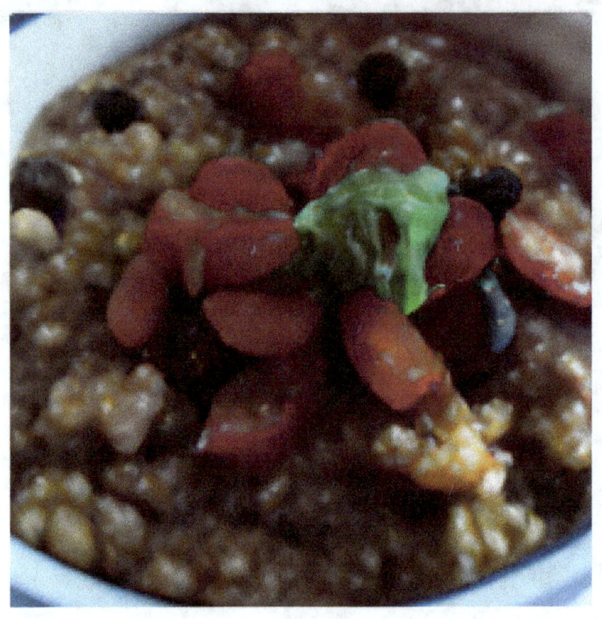

Ingredients:

- 1/2 cup rolled oats
- 1 cup vegetable broth
- Kalamata olives, sliced
- Cherry tomatoes, halved

Toppings:

Feta cheese crumbles, fresh basil, a drizzle of olive oil

Preparation:

1. Cook rolled oats in vegetable broth, incorporating sliced Kalamata olives and halved cherry tomatoes. Simmer until the oats are tender.
2. Finish with feta cheese crumbles, fresh basil, and a drizzle of olive oil.

Recipe 9. Maple Pecan Pie Oatmeal

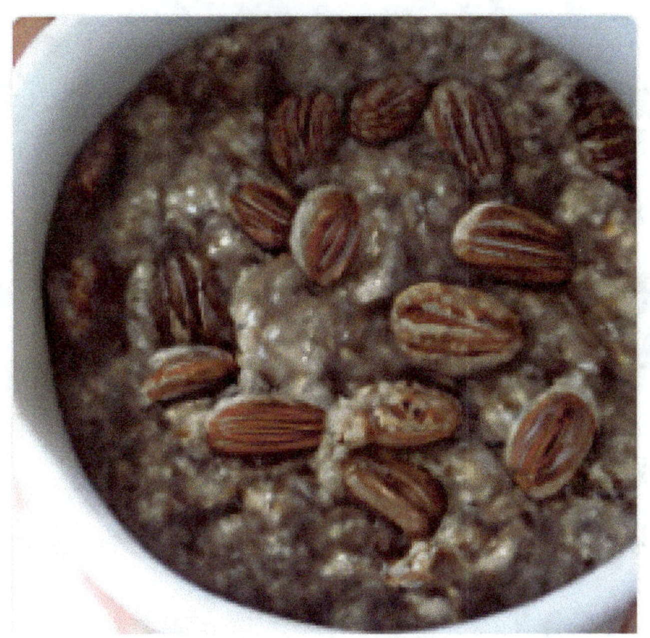

Ingredients:

- 1/2 cup old-fashioned oats
- 1 cup almond milk
- 1 tablespoon maple syrup
- Handful of chopped pecans

Preparation:

1. Mix old-fashioned oats, almond milk, maple syrup, and chopped pecans. Cook until creamy.
2. Top with sliced peaches, a sprinkle of cinnamon, and a drizzle of maple syrup.

Toppings:

Sliced peaches, a sprinkle of cinnamon, a drizzle of maple syrup

Recipe 10. Lemon Blueberry Cheesecake Oats

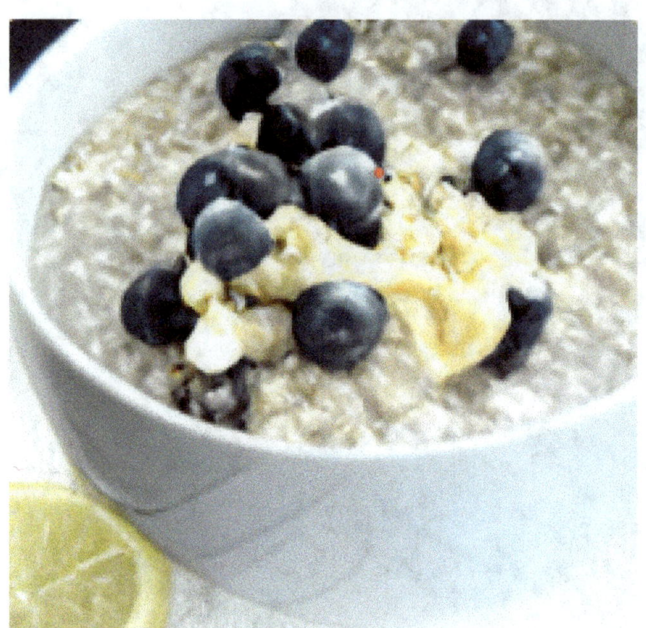

Ingredients:

- 1/2 cup rolled oats
- 1 cup almond milk
- Zest one lemon
- Handful of blueberries

Preparation:

1. Combine rolled oats, almond milk, lemon zest, and blueberries.
2. Continue cooking until the oats attain the consistency you desire. Garnish with a dollop of Greek yogurt, a drizzle of honey, and lemon slices.

Toppings:

Greek yogurt, a drizzle of honey, lemon slices

Nutrient-Packed Breakfast Parfaits

Recipe 1. Berry Almond Crunch Parfait

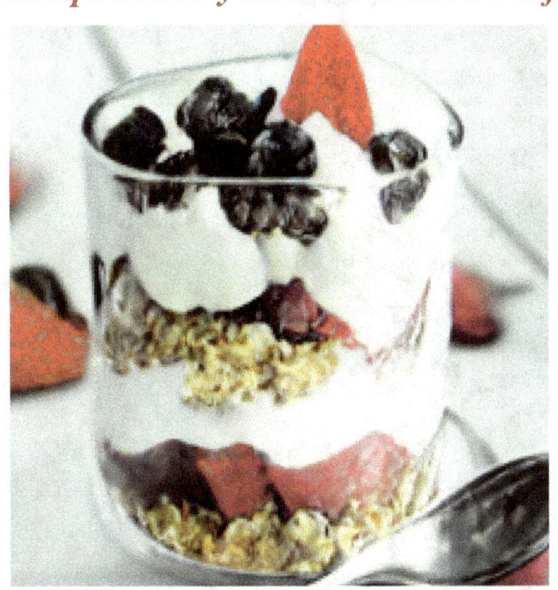

Ingredients:

- 1/2 cup Greek yogurt
- 1/4 cup granola
- 1/2 cup mixed berries (strawberries, blueberries, raspberries)
- 1 tablespoon almond butter

Preparation:

1. Layer Greek yogurt, granola, mixed berries, and almond butter in a glass.
2. Repeat for additional layers. Top with sliced almonds and finish with a drizzle of honey.

Toppings:

Sliced almonds, a drizzle of honey

Recipe 2. Tropical Mango-Coconut Paradise Parfait

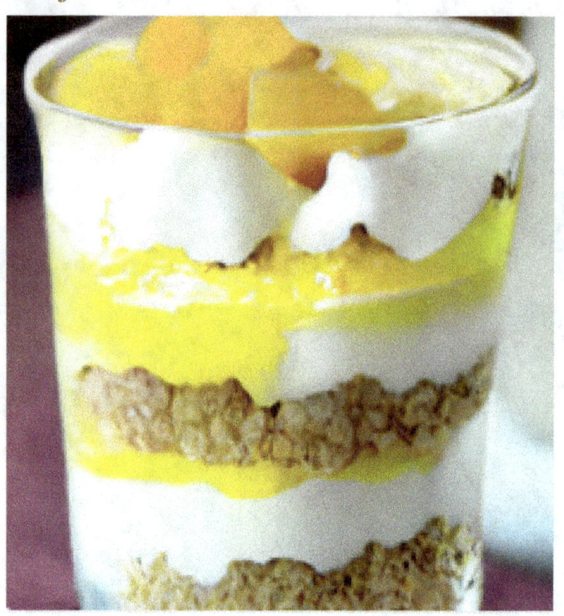

Ingredients:

- 1/2 cup coconut yogurt
- 1/2 cup mango chunks
- 2 tablespoons shredded coconut
- 1 tablespoon chia seeds

Preparation:

1. Alternate layers of coconut yogurt, mango chunks, shredded coconut, and chia seeds in a glass.
2. Garnish with kiwi slices, passion fruit seeds, and mint leaves.

Toppings:

Kiwi slices, passion fruit seeds, mint leaves

Recipe 3. Chocolate Hazelnut Indulgence Parfait

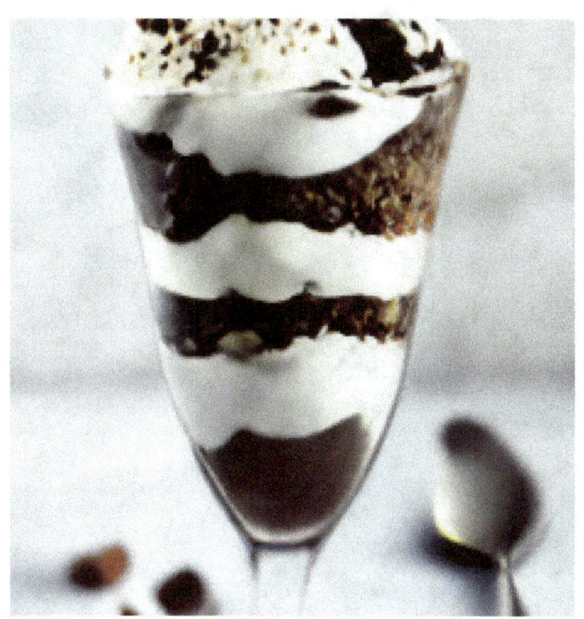

Ingredients:

- 1/2 cup chocolate-flavored Greek yogurt
- 2 tablespoons hazelnut spread
- 1/4 cup crushed hazelnuts
- 1/4 cup chocolate granola

Preparation:

1. Create layers with chocolate-flavored Greek yogurt, hazelnut spread, crushed hazelnuts, and chocolate granola in a glass.
2. Top with raspberries and dust with cocoa powder.

Toppings:

Raspberries, a dusting of cocoa powder

Recipe 4. Green Tea Matcha Bliss Parfait

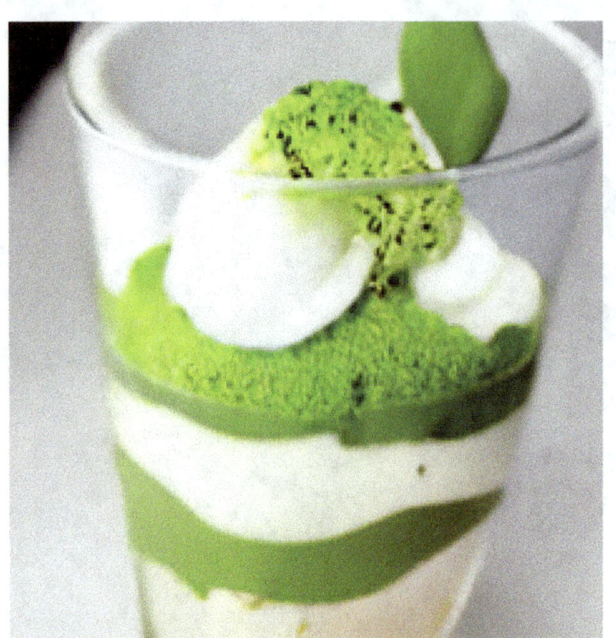

Ingredients:

- 1/2 cup vanilla yogurt
- 1 teaspoon matcha powder
- 1/4 cup sliced kiwi
- 1/4 cup green grapes, halved

Preparation:

1. Mix matcha powder into vanilla yogurt. Layer the matcha-infused yogurt with sliced kiwi and halved green grapes.
2. Top with pistachios and drizzle with agave syrup.

Toppings:

Pistachios, a drizzle of agave syrup

Recipe 5. Peanut Butter Banana Protein Parfait

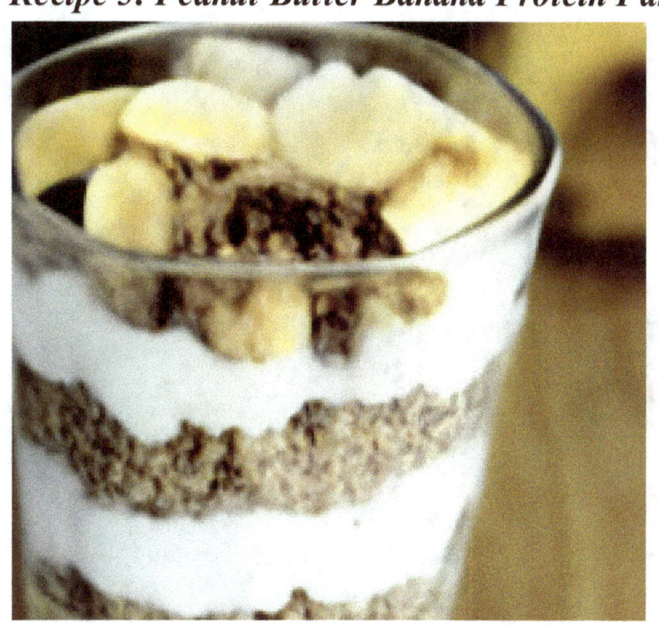

Ingredients:

- 1/2 cup vanilla Greek yogurt
- 1 tablespoon peanut butter
- 1 banana, sliced
- 2 tablespoons protein granola

Preparation:

1. Alternate layers of vanilla Greek yogurt, peanut butter, banana slices, and protein granola in a glass.
2. Garnish with chopped peanuts and a swirl of peanut butter..

Toppings:

Chopped peanuts, a swirl of peanut butter

Recipe 6. Chia Seed Pudding Berry Parfait

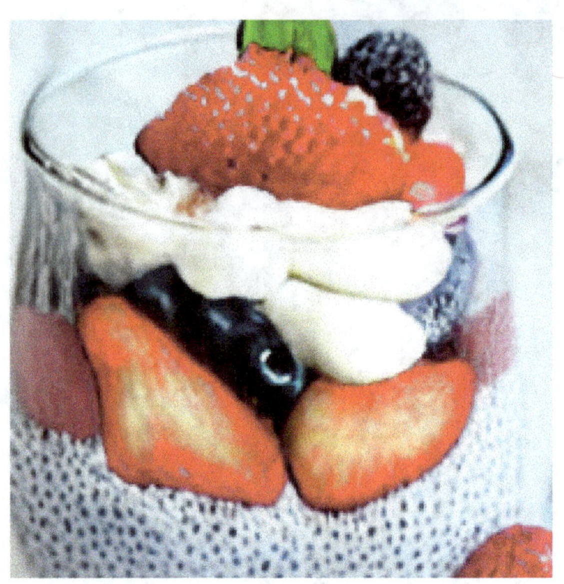

Ingredients:

- 1/4 cup chia seed pudding
- 1/2 cup mixed berries (strawberries, blueberries, raspberries)
- 1/4 cup almond yogurt
- 2 tablespoons sliced almonds

Toppings:

Fresh mint leaves, a drizzle of maple syrup

Preparation:

1. Layer chia seed pudding, mixed berries, and almond yogurt in a glass. Repeat for additional layers.
2. Top with sliced almonds, fresh mint leaves, and a drizzle of maple syrup.

Recipe 7. Peach Melba Yogurt Parfait

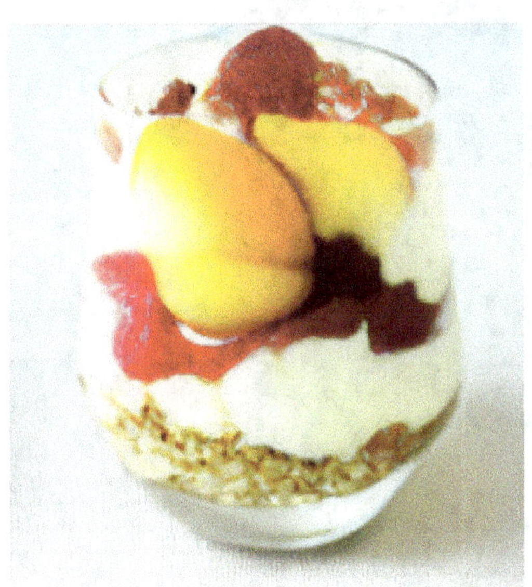

Ingredients:

- 1/2 cup peach-flavored yogurt
- 1/2 cup peach slices
- 1/4 cup raspberry compote
- 1/4 cup vanilla granola

Preparation:

1. Create layers with peach-flavored yogurt, peach slices, raspberry compote, and vanilla granola.

Recipe 8. Blueberry-Lemon Cheesecake Parfait

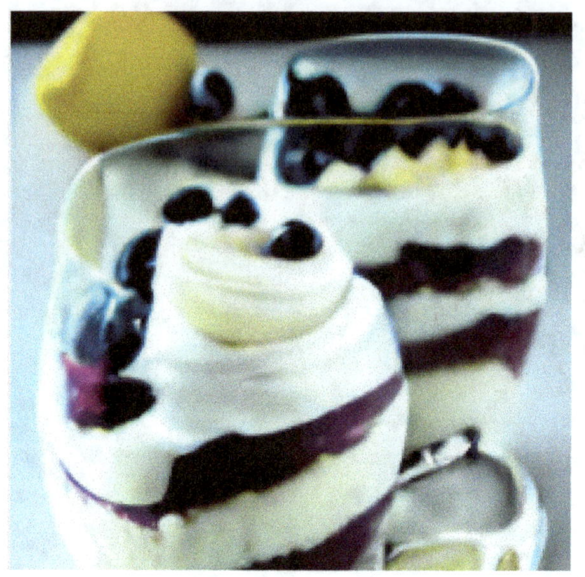

Ingredients:

- 1/2 cup lemon-flavored Greek yogurt
- 1/2 cup blueberries
- 2 tablespoons granola
- 1 tablespoon cream cheese

Preparation:

1. Layer lemon-flavored Greek yogurt, blueberries, granola, and small dollops of cream cheese in a glass.
2. Garnish with lemon zest and a drizzle of honey.

Recipe 9. Cinnamon Apple Pie Parfait

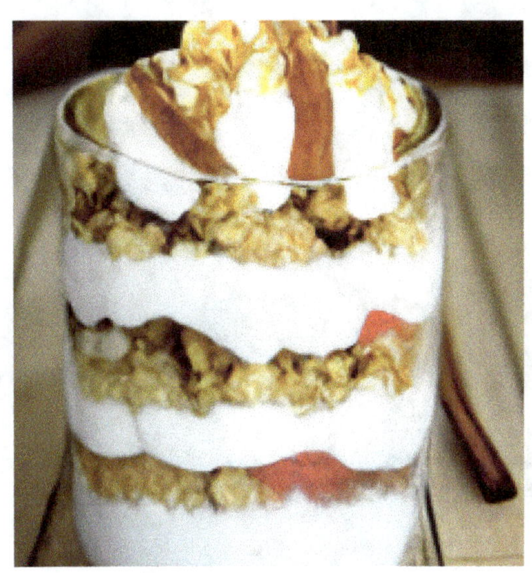

Ingredients:

- 1/2 cup cinnamon-flavored yogurt
- 1/2 cup diced apples (cooked with cinnamon)
- 1/4 cup crushed cinnamon granola
- 1 tablespoon almond butter

Preparation:

1. Create layers with cinnamon-flavored yogurt, diced apples, crushed cinnamon granola, and almond butter.
2. Top with chopped walnuts and a sprinkle of cinnamon.

Recipe 10. Mocha Banana Espresso Parfait

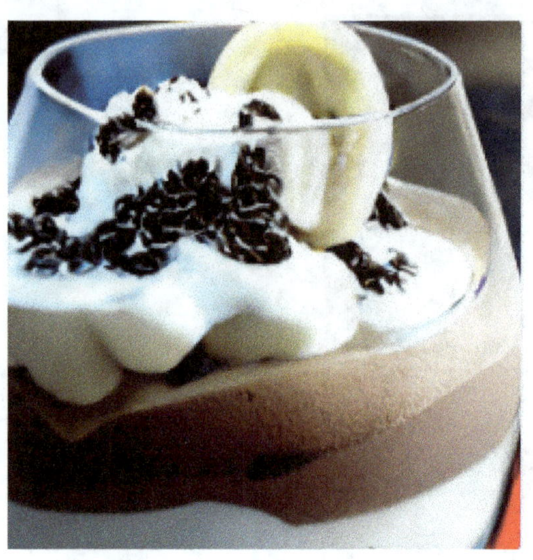

Ingredients:

- 1/2 cup mocha-flavored yogurt
- 1 banana, sliced
- 2 tablespoons espresso granola
- 1 tablespoon chocolate syrup

Preparation:

1. Layer mocha-flavored yogurt, banana slices, espresso granola, and drizzles of chocolate syrup.
2. Garnish with coffee beans and a dusting of cocoa powder.

Chapter 4
Lunchtime Favorites
Vibrant Salad Creations

Recipe 1. Mediterranean Quinoa Salad

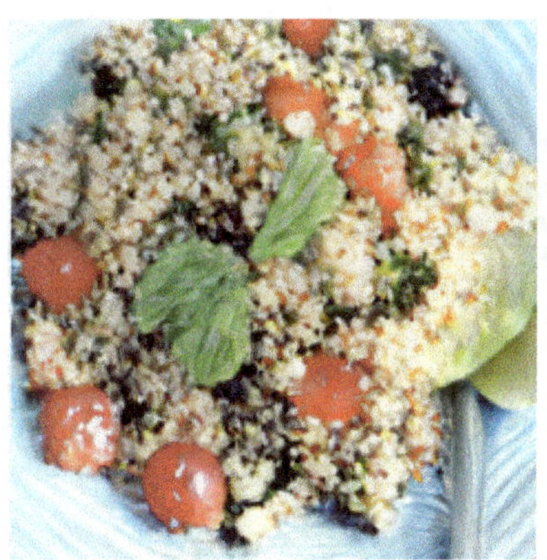

Ingredients:

- 1 cup cooked quinoa
- Cherry tomatoes, halved
- Cucumber, diced
- Kalamata olives, sliced
- Red onion, finely chopped
- Feta cheese, crumbled
- Fresh parsley, chopped

Dressings:

Olive oil

Lemon juice

Dijon mustard

Garlic, minced

Salt and pepper to taste

Preparation:

1. In a large bowl, combine cooked quinoa, cherry tomatoes, cucumber, Kalamata olives, red onion, feta cheese, and fresh parsley.
2. Whisk together olive oil, lemon juice, Dijon mustard, minced garlic, salt, and pepper in a separate bowl.
3. Infuse the salad with the dressing, achieving a homogenous blend.

Recipe 2. Asian-Inspired Sesame Ginger Salad

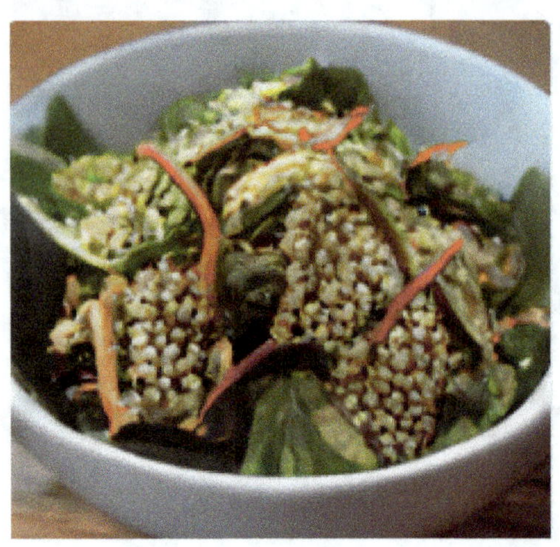

Ingredients:

- Mixed greens
- Shredded cabbage
- Carrots, julienned
- Edamame, steamed
- Red bell pepper, thinly sliced
- Sesame seeds
- Green onions, chopped

Dressings:

Soy sauce
Rice vinegar
Sesame oil
Fresh ginger, grated
Honey
Garlic powder

Preparation:

1. In a large salad bowl, combine mixed greens, shredded cabbage, julienned carrots, steamed edamame, sliced red bell pepper, sesame seeds, and chopped green onions.
2. In a small bowl, whisk together soy sauce, rice vinegar, sesame oil, grated fresh ginger, honey, and a dash of garlic powder.
3. Infuse the salad with the dressing, achieving a homogenous blend. **56**

Recipe 3. Southwest Quinoa Bowl

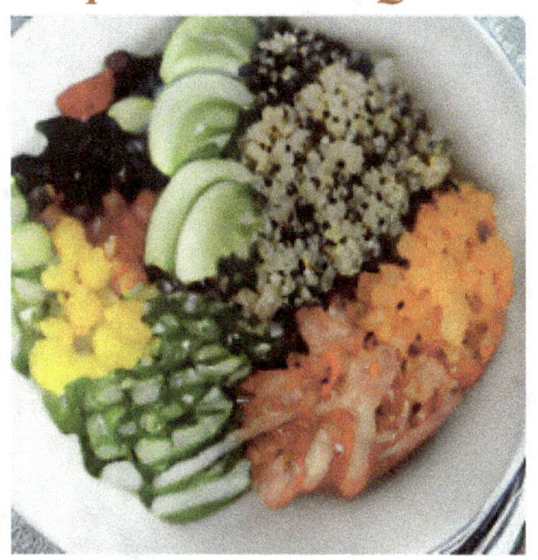

Ingredients:

- 1 cup cooked quinoa
- Black beans, rinsed and drained
- Corn kernels, fresh or roasted
- Avocado, diced
- Cherry tomatoes, halved
- Red onion, finely chopped
- Cilantro, chopped
- Lime wedges

Dressings:

Olive oil
Lime juice
Ground cumin
Chili powder
Salt and pepper to taste

Preparation:

1. Combine cooked quinoa, black beans, corn kernels, diced avocado, cherry tomatoes, red onion, and cilantro in a large bowl.
2. In a separate bowl, whisk together olive oil, lime juice, ground cumin, chili powder, salt, and pepper.
3. Apply the dressing in a fine stream over the salad, then toss to ensure even distribution. Serve with lime wedges on the side.

Recipe 4. Strawberry Spinach Salad with Balsamic Vinaigrette

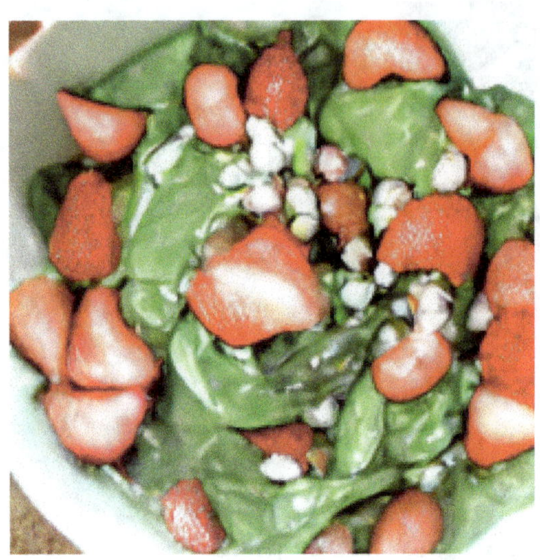

Ingredients:

- Baby spinach leaves
- Fresh strawberries, sliced
- Goat cheese, crumbled
- Candied pecans
- Red onion, thinly sliced

Dressings:

Balsamic vinegar

Olive oil

Dijon mustard

Honey

Salt and pepper to taste

Preparation:

1. In a large salad bowl, combine baby spinach leaves, sliced fresh strawberries, crumbled goat cheese, candied pecans, and thinly sliced red onion.
2. In a small bowl, whisk together balsamic vinegar, olive oil, Dijon mustard, honey, salt, and pepper. Dress the salad with a drizzle of the sauce, incorporating it delicately.

Recipe 5. Chickpea and Avocado Caesar Salad

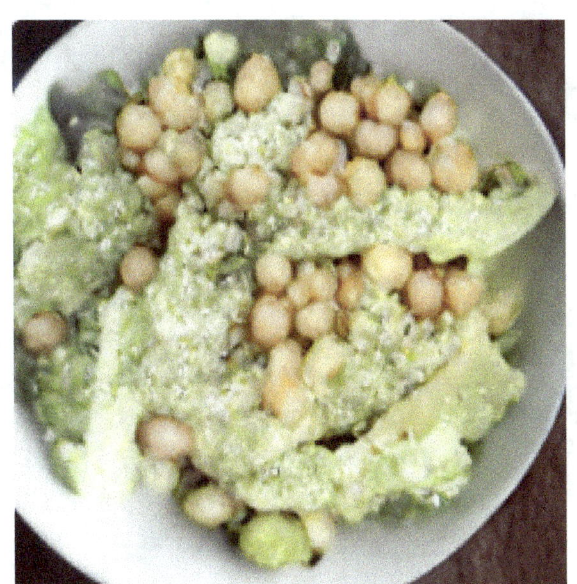

Ingredients:

- Romaine lettuce, chopped
- Chickpeas, drained and rinsed
- Cherry tomatoes, halved
- Avocado, sliced
- Parmesan cheese, shaved

Dressings:

Anchovy paste
Garlic, minced
Dijon mustard
Lemon juice
Olive oil
Salt and pepper to taste

Preparation:

1. In a large bowl, combine chopped romaine lettuce, chickpeas, cherry tomatoes, avocado slices, and shaved Parmesan cheese.
2. In a blender, blend Greek yogurt, anchovy paste, minced garlic, Dijon mustard, lemon juice, olive oil, salt, and pepper until smooth.
3. Lightly dress the salad with Caesar dressing, folding gently to distribute.

Recipe 6. Roasted Vegetable Quinoa Salad

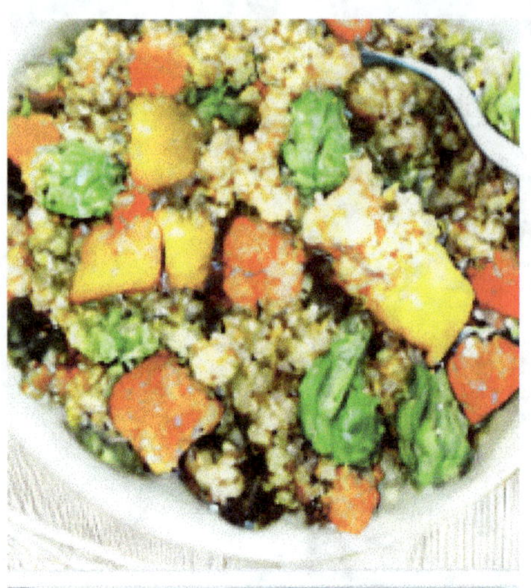

Ingredients:

- 1 cup cooked quinoa
- Bell peppers, assorted colors, sliced
- Zucchini, sliced
- Cherry tomatoes
- Red onion, thinly sliced
- Feta cheese, crumbled
- Fresh basil, chopped

Dressings:

Balsamic vinegar

Olive oil

Honey

Salt and pepper to taste

Preparation:

1. Combine cooked quinoa, sliced bell peppers, zucchini, cherry tomatoes, red onion, feta cheese, and fresh basil in a large bowl.
2. In a small saucepan, simmer balsamic vinegar, olive oil, honey, salt, and pepper until it forms a glaze.
3. Drizzle the balsamic glaze over the salad and toss gently.

Recipe 7. Tex-Mex Taco Salad Bowl

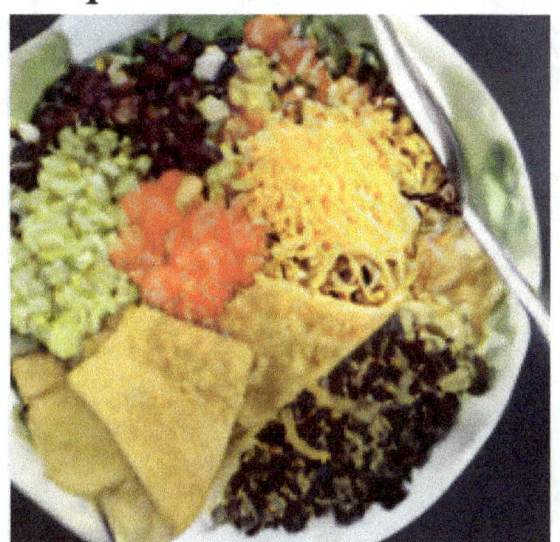

Ingredients:

- Mixed greens
- Ground turkey or black beans for a vegetarian option
- Cherry tomatoes, halved
- Avocado, diced
- Corn kernels, fresh or roasted
- Shredded cheddar cheese
- Tortilla strips

Dressings:

Greek yogurt
Taco seasoning
Lime juice
Salt and pepper to taste

Preparation:

1. In a large bowl, layer mixed greens, cooked ground turkey or black beans, cherry tomatoes, diced avocado, corn kernels, shredded cheddar cheese, and tortilla strips.
2. In a small bowl, whisk together Greek yogurt, taco seasoning, lime juice, salt, and pepper.
3. Drizzle the taco dressing over the salad and toss gently.

Recipe 8. Caprese Salad with Pesto Drizzle

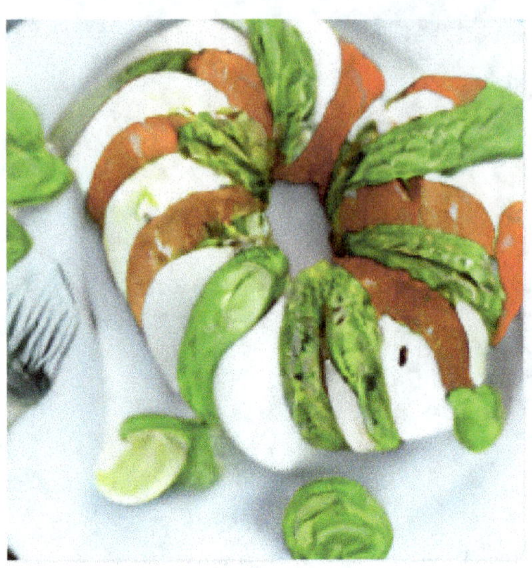

Ingredients:

- Fresh mozzarella, sliced
- Tomatoes, sliced
- Fresh basil leaves
- Balsamic glaze
- Pine nuts, toasted

Dressings:

Fresh basil

Parmesan cheese, grated

Garlic, minced

Pine nuts

Olive oil

Salt and pepper to taste

Preparation:

1. Arrange slices of fresh mozzarella, tomatoes, and fresh basil leaves on a serving platter. Drizzle with balsamic glaze.
2. In a blender, blend fresh basil, grated Parmesan cheese, minced garlic, pine nuts, olive oil, salt, and pepper until it forms a pesto.
3. Drizzle the pesto over the Caprese salad and sprinkle with toasted pine nuts.

Recipe 9. Harvest Quinoa Salad with Maple Dijon Dressing

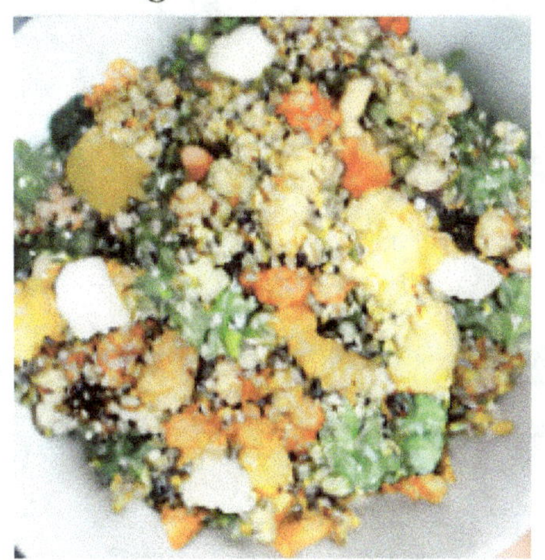

Ingredients:

- 1 cup cooked quinoa
- Butternut squash, diced and roasted
- Brussels sprouts, halved and roasted
- Dried cranberries
- Pecans, toasted
- Goat cheese, crumbled

Dressings:

Olive oil

Balsamic vinegar

Dijon mustard

Maple syrup

Salt and pepper to taste

Preparation:

1. Combine cooked quinoa, roasted butternut squash, roasted Brussels sprouts, dried cranberries, toasted pecans, and crumbled goat cheese in a large bowl.
2. Prepare a vinaigrette by whisking olive oil, balsamic vinegar, Dijon mustard, maple syrup, salt, and pepper in a small bowl.
3. Infuse the salad with the dressing, achieving a homogenous blend.

Recipe 10. Avocado and Black Bean Fiesta Salad

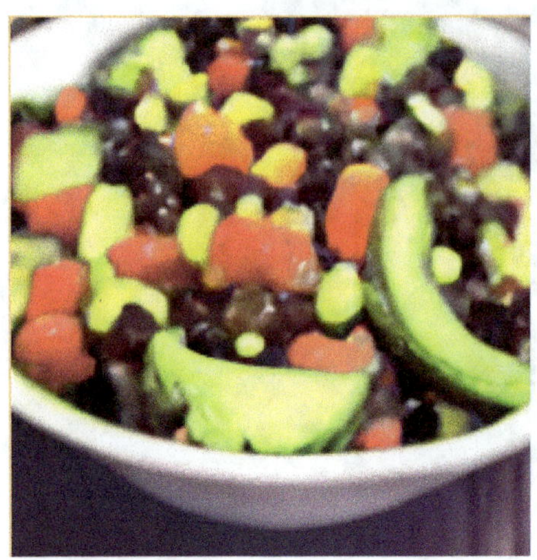

Ingredients:

- Mixed greens
- Black beans, rinsed and drained
- Corn kernels, fresh or roasted
- Cherry tomatoes, halved
- Avocado, diced
- Red onion, finely chopped
- Cilantro, chopped

Dressings:

Lime juice
Olive oil
Fresh cilantro, chopped
Garlic, minced
Honey
Salt and pepper to taste

Preparation:

1. Layer mixed greens, black beans, corn kernels, cherry tomatoes, diced avocado, red onion, and chopped cilantro in a large salad bowl.
2. In a small bowl, whisk together lime juice, olive oil, chopped cilantro, minced garlic, honey, salt, and pepper.
3. Drizzle the cilantro lime vinaigrette over the salad and toss gently.

Hearty Plant-Based Soups

Recipe 1. Tuscan White Bean and Kale Soup

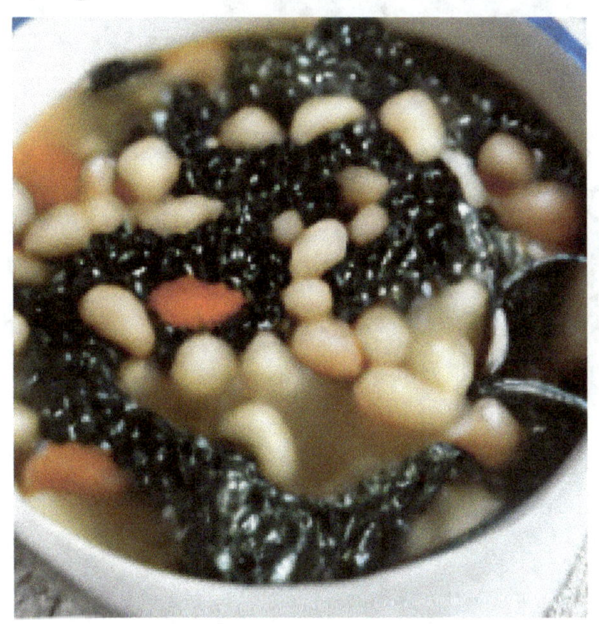

Ingredients:

- Cannellini beans, cooked
- Kale, chopped
- Carrots, diced
- Celery, sliced
- Garlic, minced
- Vegetable broth
- Italian herbs (rosemary, thyme, oregano)
- Salt and pepper to taste

Preparation:

1. In a large pot, sauté garlic, carrots, and celery until softened.
2. Add cooked cannellini beans, chopped kale, vegetable broth, and Italian herbs.
3. Simmer until the kale is tender. Season with salt and pepper as much as you want.

Recipe 2. Lentil and Vegetable Curry Soup

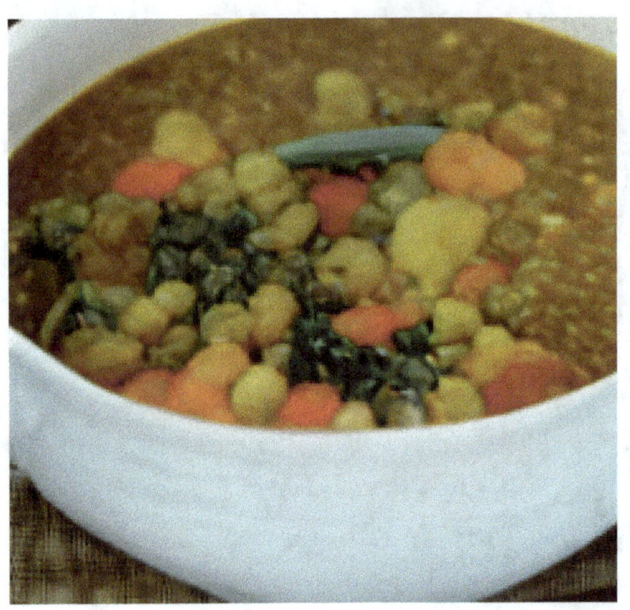

Ingredients:

- Red lentils, rinsed
- Sweet potatoes, diced
- Cauliflower, chopped
- Onion, finely chopped
- Coconut milk
- Curry powder
- Turmeric
- Vegetable broth
- Salt and pepper to taste

Preparation:

1. Sauté onion until translucent.
2. Add sweet potatoes, cauliflower, red lentils, curry powder, turmeric, and vegetable broth.
3. Simmer until lentils are cooked. Stir in coconut milk and season with salt and pepper.

Recipe 3. Moroccan Chickpea and Vegetable Stew

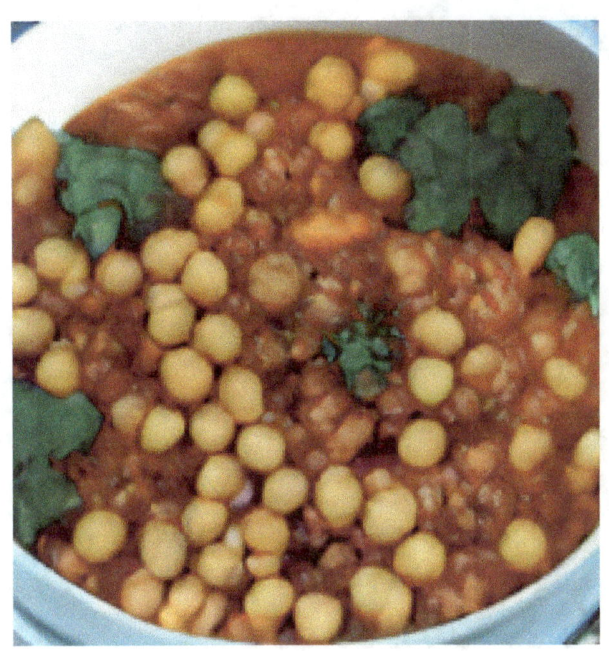

Ingredients:

- Chickpeas, cooked
- Eggplant, diced
- Bell peppers, chopped
- Zucchini, sliced
- Tomatoes, diced
- Cumin, coriander, paprika
- Vegetable broth
- Fresh cilantro, chopped
- Lemon wedges

Preparation:

1. In a pot, combine chickpeas, eggplant, bell peppers, zucchini, tomatoes, cumin, coriander, paprika, and vegetable broth.
2. Simmer until vegetables are tender. Garnish with fresh cilantro and serve with lemon wedges.

Recipe 4. Butternut Squash and Apple Soup

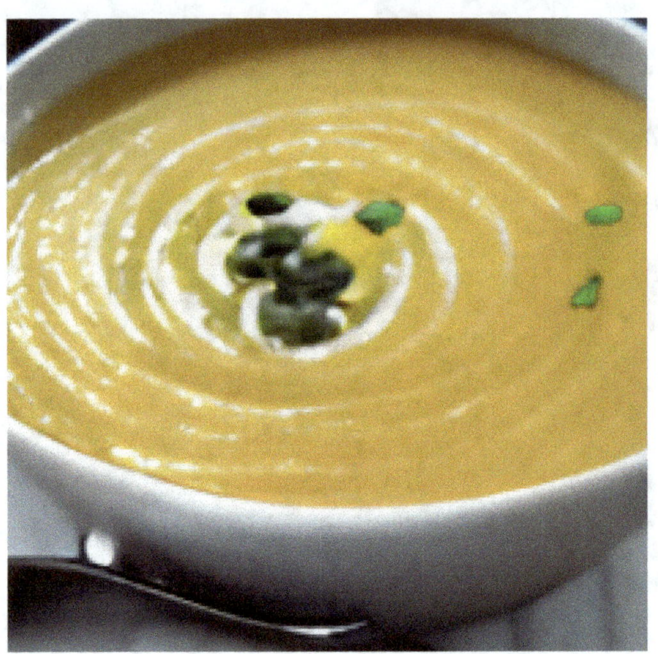

Ingredients:

- Butternut squash, peeled and cubed
- Apples, peeled and diced
- Onion, chopped
- Vegetable broth
- Coconut milk
- Nutmeg, cinnamon
- Maple syrup
- Salt and pepper to taste

Preparation:

1. Sauté onion until translucent. Add butternut squash, apples, vegetable broth, coconut milk, nutmeg, cinnamon, and maple syrup.
2. Simmer until the squash and apples are soft. Blend until smooth and season with salt and pepper.

Recipe 5. Quinoa Minestrone Soup

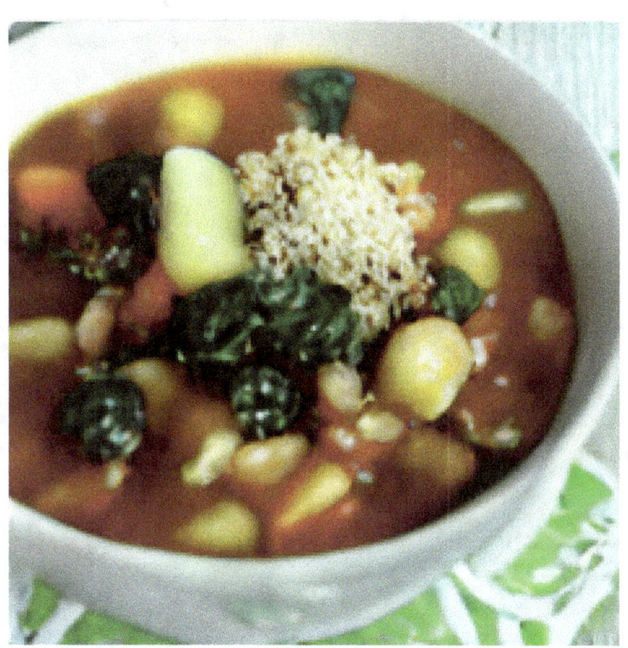

Ingredients:

- Quinoa, rinsed
- Cannellini beans, cooked
- Tomatoes, diced
- Carrots, sliced
- Spinach, chopped
- Vegetable broth
- Italian seasoning
- Garlic powder
- Salt and pepper to taste

Preparation:

1. In a pot, combine quinoa, cannellini beans, tomatoes, carrots, spinach, vegetable broth, Italian seasoning, and garlic powder.
2. Simmer until the quinoa is cooked. Season with salt and pepper.

Recipe 6. *Thai Coconut and Vegetable Noodle Soup*

Ingredients:

- Rice noodles, cooked
- Broccoli, florets
- Mushrooms, sliced
- Bell peppers, thinly sliced
- Coconut milk
- Thai red curry paste
- Lemongrass, minced
- Vegetable broth
- Soy sauce
- Lime wedges

Preparation:

1. In a pot, combine broccoli, mushrooms, bell peppers, coconut milk, Thai red curry paste, lemongrass, vegetable broth, and soy sauce.

2. Simmer until vegetables are tender. Serve over cooked rice noodles and garnish with lime wedges.

Recipe 7. Black Bean and Corn Chili

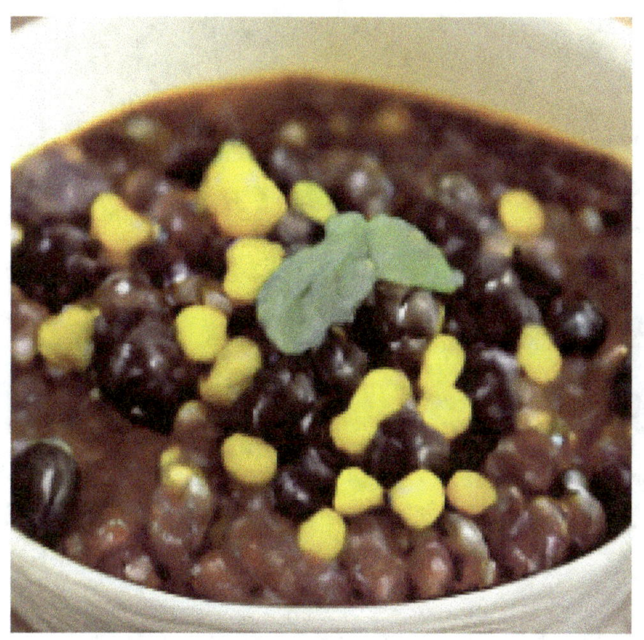

Ingredients:

- Black beans, cooked
- Corn kernels
- Bell peppers, diced
- Onion, chopped
- Tomatoes, diced
- Chili powder, cumin, smoked paprika
- Vegetable broth
- Cilantro, chopped
- Avocado slices

Preparation:

1. Sauté onion until translucent. Add black beans, corn, bell peppers, tomatoes, chili powder, cumin, smoked paprika, and vegetable broth.
2. Simmer until flavors meld. Finished with fragrant cilantro and accompanied by avocado slices.

Recipe 8. Wild Rice and Mushroom Soup

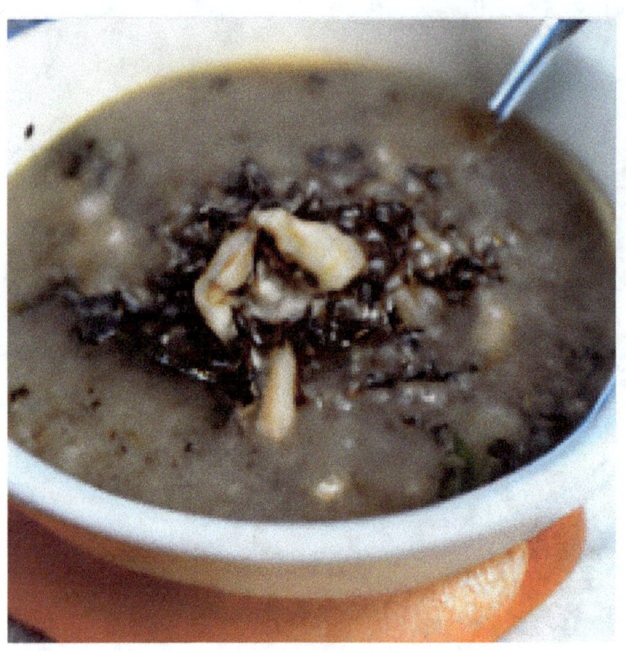

Ingredients:

- Wild rice, cooked
- Mushrooms, sliced
- Carrots, diced
- Celery, sliced
- Onion, chopped
- Vegetable broth
- Thyme, rosemary
- Almond milk
- Salt and pepper to taste

Preparation:

1. Sauté onion until translucent. Add mushrooms, carrots, celery, wild rice, vegetable broth, thyme, and rosemary.
2. Simmer until vegetables are tender. Stir in almond milk and season with salt and pepper.

Recipe 9. Roasted Red Pepper and Tomato Basil Soup

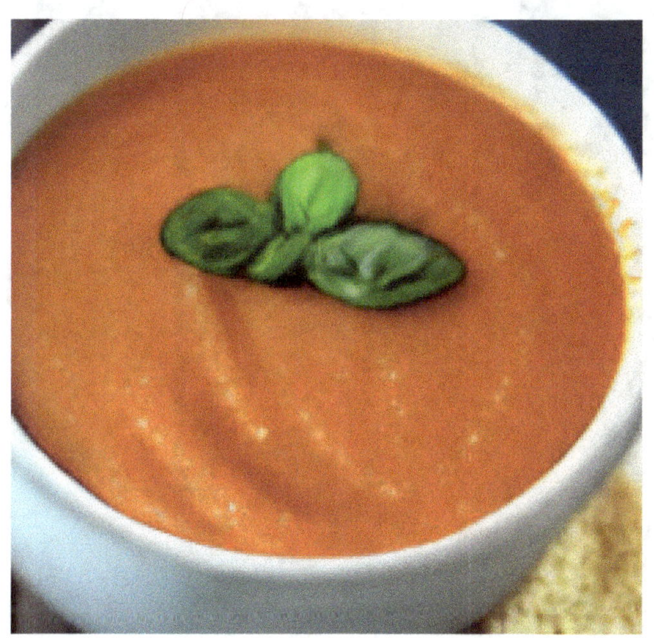

Ingredients:

- Roasted red peppers, chopped
- Tomatoes, diced
- Onion, chopped
- Garlic, minced
- Vegetable broth
- Basil, fresh or dried
- Balsamic vinegar
- Salt and pepper to taste

Preparation:

1. In a pot, combine roasted red peppers, tomatoes, onion, garlic, vegetable broth, and basil. Simmer until vegetables are soft.
2. Blend until smooth, stir in balsamic vinegar, and season with salt and pepper.

Recipe 10. Spinach and White Bean Tortellini Soup

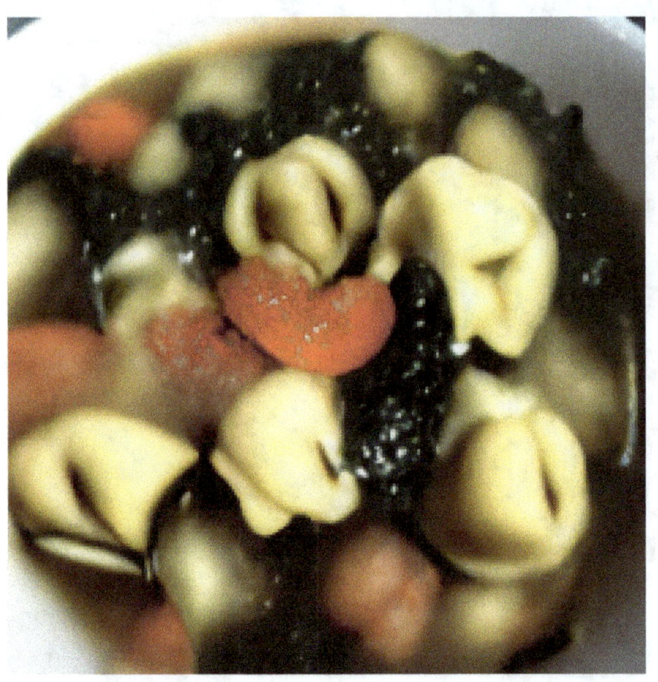

Ingredients:

- Cheese or vegan spinach tortellini
- White beans, cooked
- Spinach, chopped
- Tomatoes, diced
- Vegetable broth
- Italian herbs
- Garlic powder
- Parmesan or vegan cheese, grated

Preparation:

1. Cook tortellini according to package instructions. In a pot, combine cooked tortellini, white beans, spinach, tomatoes, vegetable broth, Italian herbs, and garlic powder.
2. Simmer until the tortellini is heated through. Serve topped with grated Parmesan or vegan cheese.

Nourishing Buddha Bowls

Recipe 1. Quinoa and Roasted Vegetable Bliss Bowl

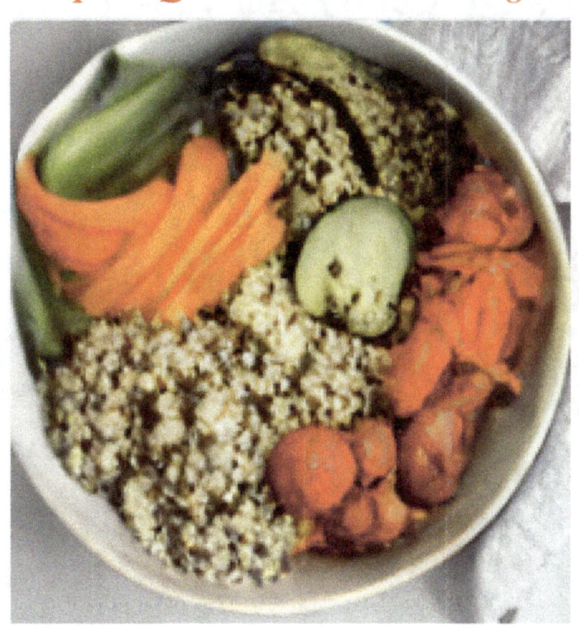

Ingredients:

- Tri-color quinoa, cooked
- Roasted sweet potatoes, carrots, and Brussels sprouts
- Chickpeas, roasted
- Avocado slices
- Kale, massaged
- Tahini dressing

Preparation:

1. Layer cooked quinoa with a medley of roasted sweet potatoes, carrots, Brussels sprouts, and chickpeas.
2. Add avocado slices and massaged kale. Drizzle with tahini dressing for a creamy finish.

Recipe 2. Teriyaki Tofu and Edamame Power Bowl

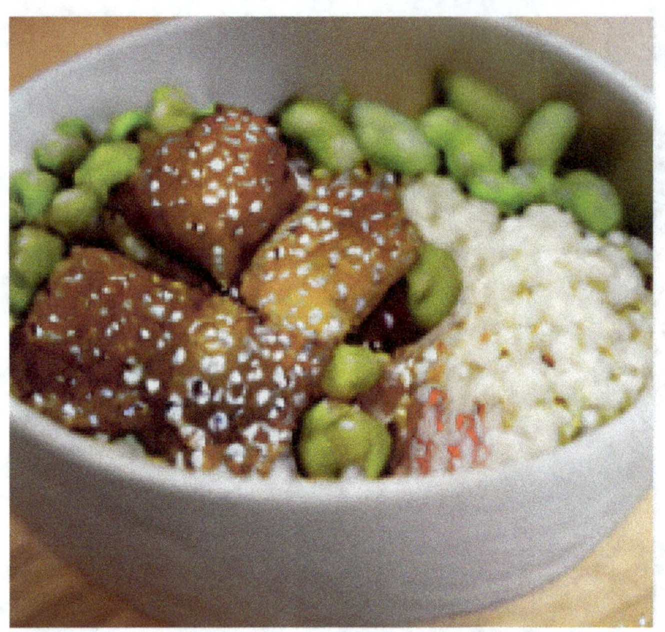

Ingredients:

- Brown rice, cooked
- Teriyaki tofu, cubed
- Edamame, steamed
- Shredded red cabbage
- Sliced cucumbers
- Sesame seeds
- Teriyaki sauce

Preparation:

1. Arrange cooked brown rice with teriyaki tofu, steamed edamame, shredded red cabbage, and sliced cucumbers.
2. Sprinkle with sesame seeds and drizzle with teriyaki sauce for an umami-packed experience.

Recipe 3. Mediterranean Chickpea and Quinoa Bowl

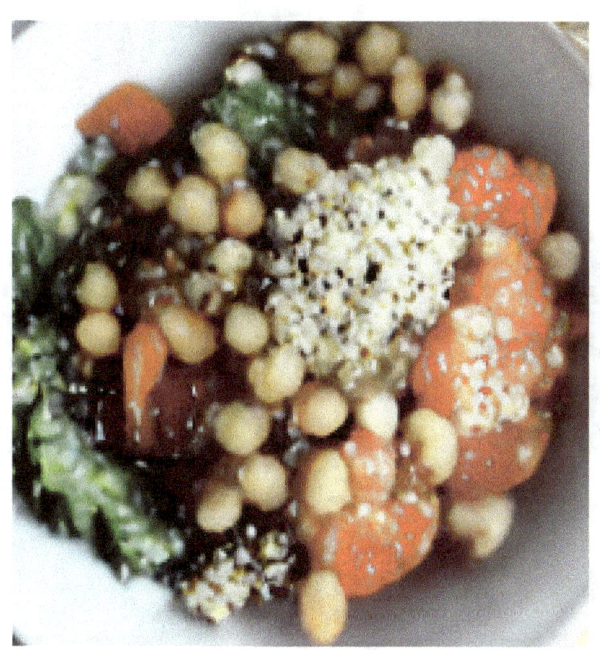

Ingredients:

- Quinoa, cooked
- Chickpeas, seasoned and roasted
- Cherry tomatoes, halved
- Cucumber, diced
- Kalamata olives, sliced
- Red onion, finely chopped
- Feta cheese, crumbled
- Greek dressing

Preparation:

1. Combine cooked quinoa with seasoned and roasted chickpeas, cherry tomatoes, diced cucumber, sliced Kalamata olives, finely chopped red onion, and crumbled feta cheese.
2. Finish with a touch of Greek dressing for a Mediterranean flair.

Recipe 4. Spicy Black Bean and Avocado Fiesta Bowl

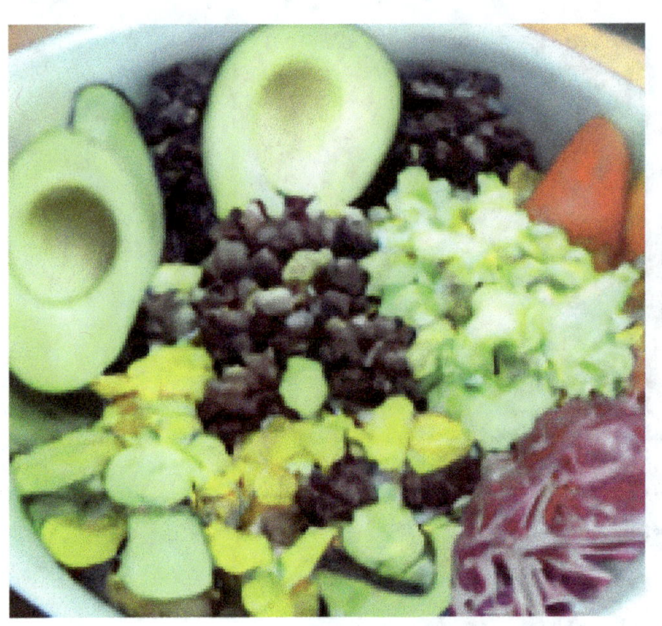

Ingredients:

- Black beans, seasoned and cooked
- Brown rice, cooked
- Avocado, sliced
- Corn kernels, fresh or roasted
- Red onion, finely chopped
- Fresh cilantro, chopped
- Lime wedges
- Spicy salsa

Preparation:

1. Layer seasoned black beans with cooked brown rice, sliced avocado, corn kernels, finely chopped red onion, and chopped fresh cilantro.

2. Serve with lime wedges and a dollop of spicy salsa for a fiesta in every bite.

Recipe 5. Asian-Inspired Forbidden Rice and Vegetable Bowl

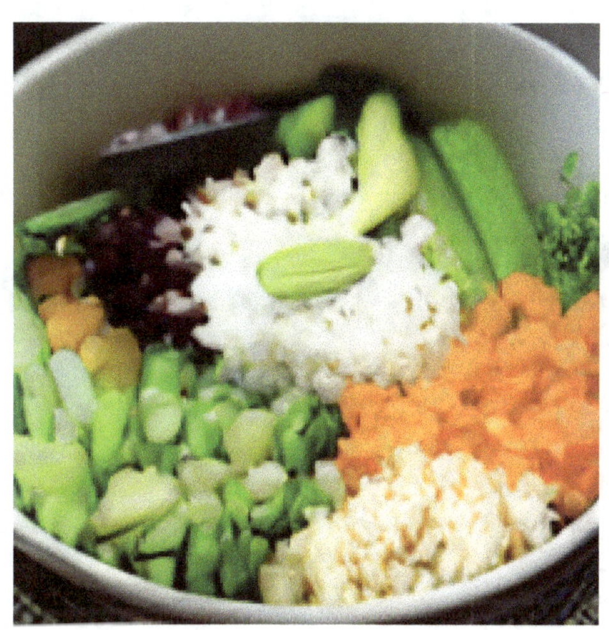

Ingredients:

- Forbidden rice, cooked
- Stir-fried tofu
- Broccoli florets, steamed
- Shredded carrots
- Snap peas, blanched
- Green onions, sliced
- Soy-ginger dressing

Preparation:

1. Combine cooked Forbidden rice with stir-fried tofu, steamed broccoli florets, shredded carrots, blanched snap peas, and sliced green onions.
2. Drizzle with soy-ginger dressing for an Asian-inspired sensation.

Recipe 6. Roasted Cauliflower and Hummus Quinoa Bowl

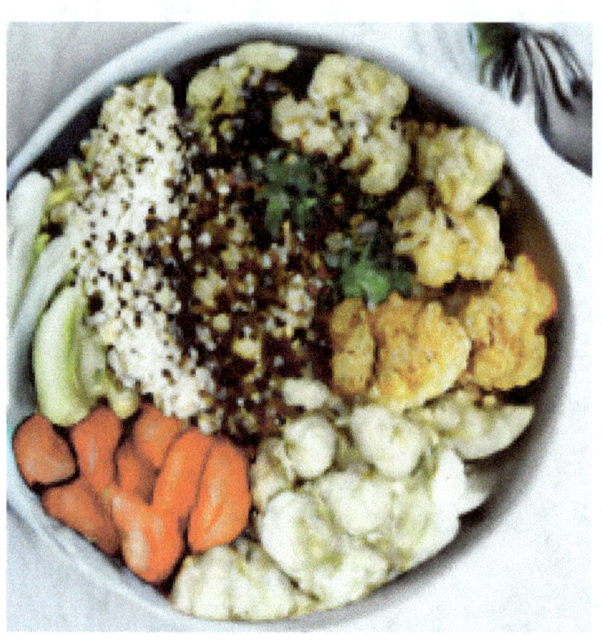

Ingredients:

- Quinoa, cooked
- Roasted cauliflower florets
- Hummus
- Cherry tomatoes, halved
- Cucumber, sliced
- Red pepper flakes
- Lemon-tahini dressing

Preparation:

1. Layer cooked quinoa with roasted cauliflower florets, a generous dollop of hummus, halved cherry tomatoes, and sliced cucumber.
2. Sprinkle with red pepper flakes and drizzle with lemon-tahini dressing for a delightful combination.

Recipe 7. Pesto Pasta and Sun-Dried Tomato Delight Bowl

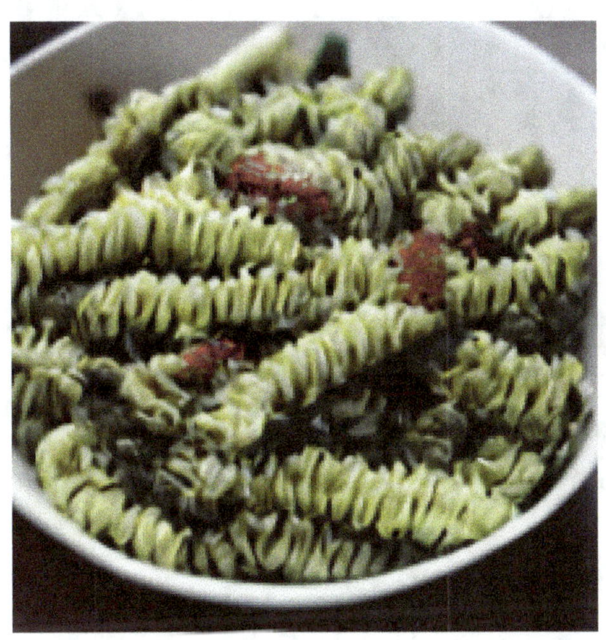

Ingredients:

- Whole wheat pasta, cooked
- Pesto sauce
- Sun-dried tomatoes, sliced
- Artichoke hearts, quartered
- Baby spinach leaves
- Pine nuts, toasted
- Balsamic glaze

Preparation:

1. Combine cooked whole wheat pasta with pesto sauce, sliced sun-dried tomatoes, quartered artichoke hearts, baby spinach leaves, and toasted pine nuts.
2. Drizzle with balsamic glaze for a Mediterranean-inspired delight.

Recipe 8. Sweet Potato and Black Rice Harvest Bowl

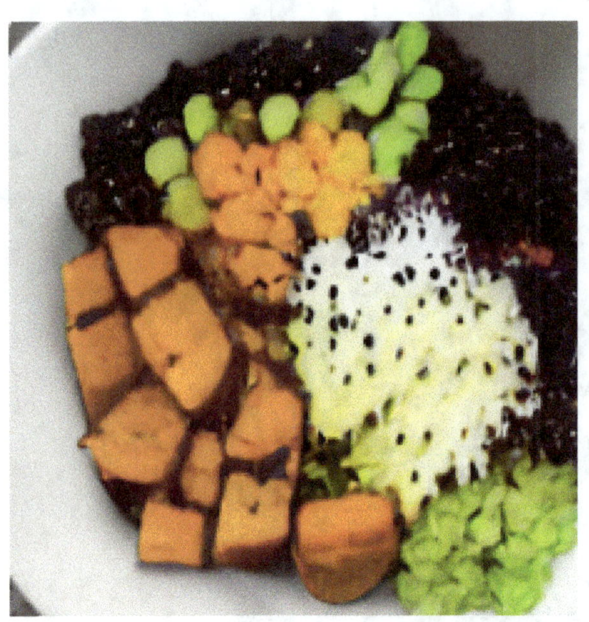

Ingredients:

- Black rice, cooked
- Roasted sweet potatoes
- Sautéed kale
- Pomegranate seeds
- Toasted pecans, chopped
- Maple-tahini dressing

Preparation:

1. Layer cooked black rice with roasted sweet potatoes, sautéed kale, pomegranate seeds, and chopped toasted pecans.
2. Drizzle with maple-tahini dressing for a harvest-inspired bowl.

Recipe 9. Falafel and Quinoa Greek Bowl

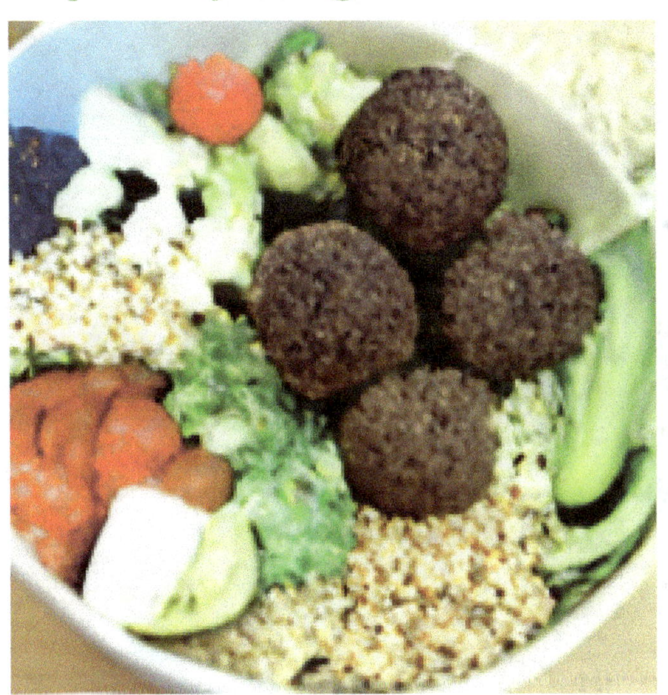

Ingredients:

- Quinoa, cooked
- Baked falafel
- Cherry tomatoes, halved
- Cucumber, diced
- Red onion, finely chopped
- Kalamata olives, sliced
- Tzatziki sauce

Preparation:

1. Combine cooked quinoa with baked falafel, halved cherry tomatoes, diced cucumber, finely chopped red onion, and sliced Kalamata olives.
2. Drizzle with tzatziki sauce for a Greek-inspired bowl.

Recipe 10. Tex-Mex Sweet Potato and Black Bean Fiesta Bowl

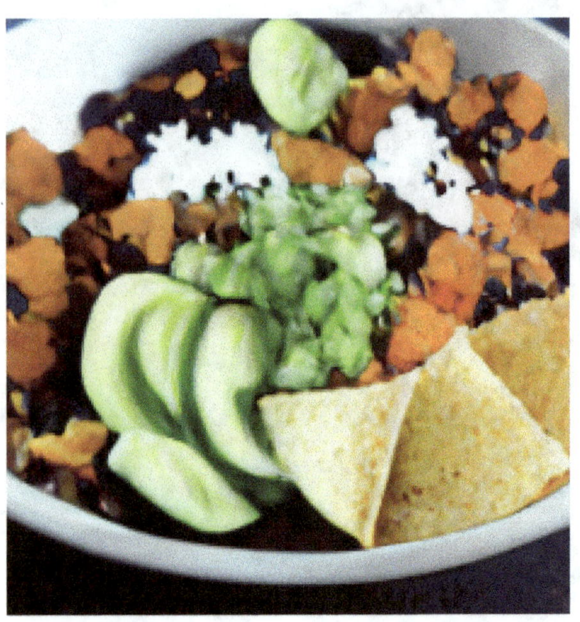

Ingredients:

- Quinoa, cooked
- Sweet potatoes, roasted
- Black beans, seasoned and cooked
- Brown rice, cooked
- Corn kernels, fresh or roasted
- Avocado, sliced
- Cilantro, chopped
- Lime wedges
- Chipotle-lime dressing

Preparation:

1. Layer roasted sweet potatoes with seasoned black beans, cooked brown rice, fresh corn kernels, sliced avocado, and chopped cilantro.
2. Serve with lime wedges and drizzle with chipotle-lime dressing for a Tex-Mex fiesta.

Chapter 5
Dinner for Healing
Plant-Powered Protein Sources

Recipe 1. Lentil and Vegetable Stew

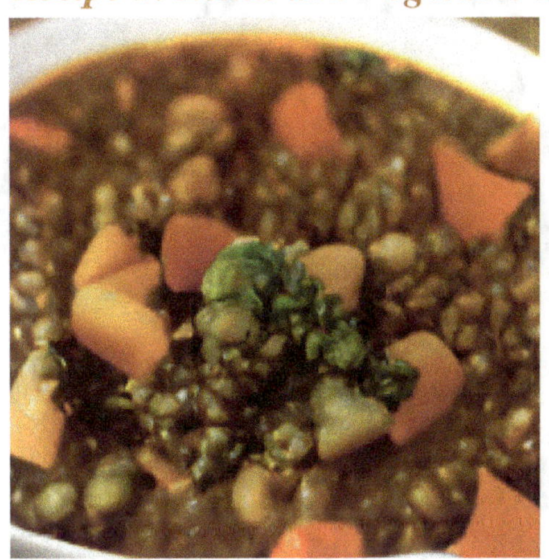

Ingredients:

- Green or brown lentils, soaked
- Carrots, diced
- Celery, sliced
- Onion, chopped
- Garlic, minced
- Vegetable broth
- Tomatoes, diced
- Spinach, chopped
- Cumin, coriander, smoked paprika
- Salt and pepper to taste

Preparation:

1. Sauté onions and garlic until fragrant. Add soaked lentils, diced carrots, sliced celery, vegetable broth, diced tomatoes, cumin, coriander, smoked paprika, salt, and pepper.
2. Simmer until lentils are tender. Stir in chopped spinach before serving.

Recipe 2. Chickpea and Spinach Curry

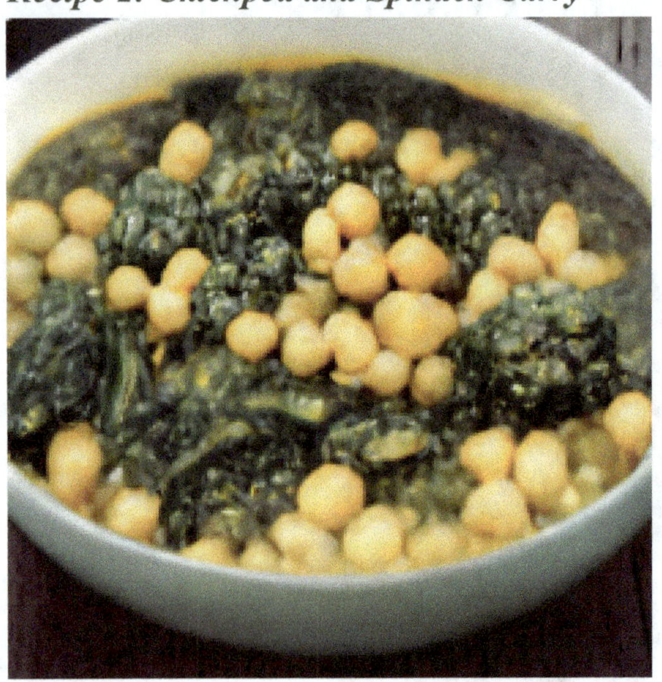

Ingredients:

- Chickpeas, cooked
- Spinach leaves
- Coconut milk
- Onion, finely chopped
- Tomatoes, pureed
- Ginger-garlic paste
- Curry powder, turmeric, cumin
- Garam masala
- Fresh cilantro, chopped
- Basmati rice (optional for serving)

Preparation:

1. Sauté chopped onion until golden brown. Add chickpeas, spinach, coconut milk, pureed tomatoes, ginger-garlic paste, curry powder, turmeric, cumin, and garam masala.
2. Simmer until flavors meld. Garnish with fresh cilantro. Serve over basmati rice if desired.

Recipe 3. Quinoa and Black Bean Stuffed Bell Peppers

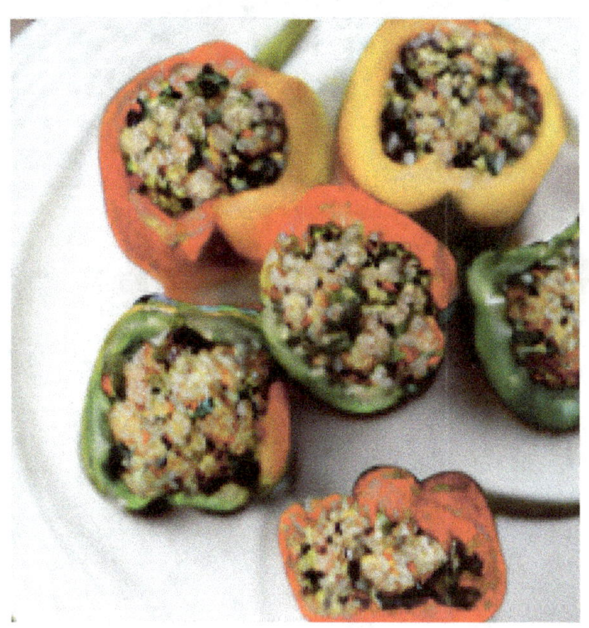

Ingredients:

- Quinoa, cooked
- Black beans, cooked
- Bell peppers, halved
- Corn kernels
- Red onion, diced
- Salsa
- Cumin, chili powder, garlic powder
- Vegan cheese (optional)

Preparation:

1. Mix cooked quinoa with black beans, corn kernels, diced red onion, salsa, cumin, chili powder, and garlic powder. Stuff the halved bell peppers with the quinoa mixture.
2. Bake until the peppers are tender. Optional: Sprinkle with vegan cheese before serving.

Recipe 4. Tofu and Vegetable Stir-Fry

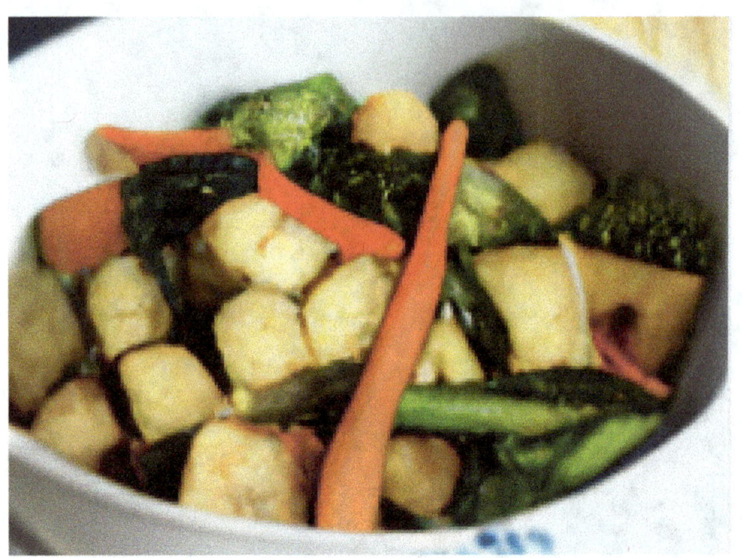

Ingredients:

- Firm tofu, cubed
- Broccoli florets
- Bell peppers, sliced
- Carrots, julienned
- Snap peas
- Ginger, minced
- Garlic, minced
- Soy sauce, sesame oil
- Rice noodles or brown rice (optional for serving)

Preparation:

1. Sauté cubed tofu until golden. Add broccoli, bell peppers, julienned carrots, snap peas, minced ginger, and minced garlic.
2. Stir in soy sauce and sesame oil. Serve over rice noodles or brown rice if desired.

Recipe 5. Mushroom and Walnut Bolognese

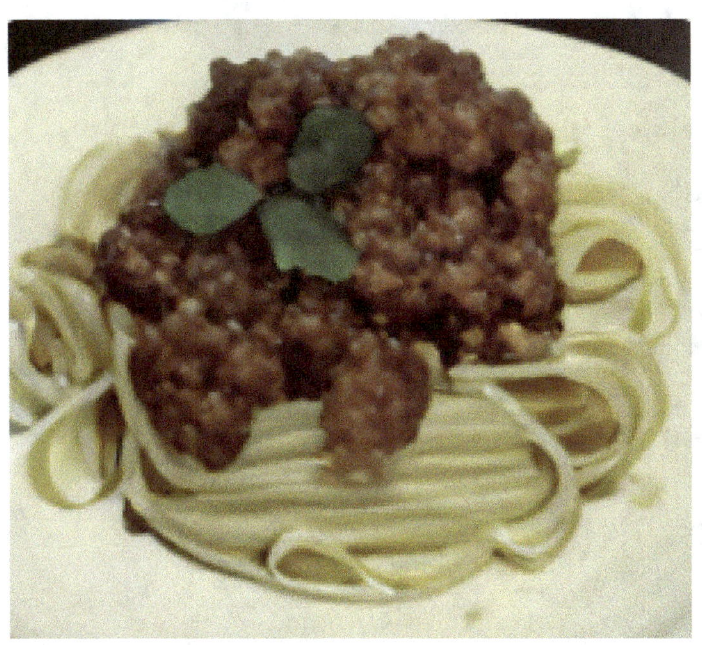

Ingredients:

- Firm tofu, cubed
- Mushrooms, finely chopped
- Walnuts, chopped
- Onion, finely chopped
- Garlic, minced
- Tomato sauce
- Red wine (optional)
- Italian herbs (oregano, basil, thyme)
- Whole wheat or gluten-free pasta

Preparation:

1. Sauté chopped onion and garlic until softened. Add finely chopped mushrooms, chopped walnuts, tomato sauce, red wine (optional), and Italian herbs.
2. Simmer until the sauce thickens. Serve over whole wheat or gluten-free pasta.

Recipe 6. Spinach and Artichoke Chickpea Pasta

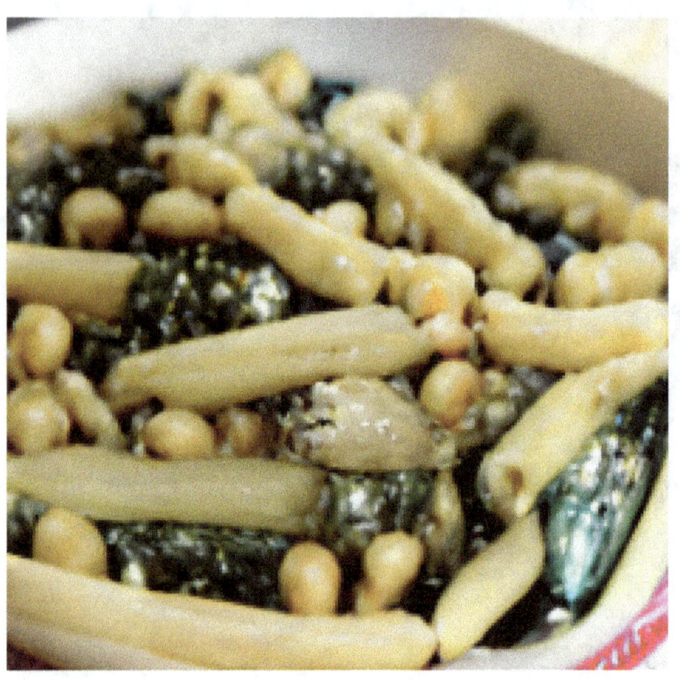

Ingredients:

- Chickpea pasta
- Spinach, chopped
- Artichoke hearts, quartered
- Cherry tomatoes, halved
- Kalamata olives, sliced
- Olive oil
- Lemon juice
- Garlic, minced
- Salt and pepper to taste

Preparation:

1. Cook chickpea pasta according to package instructions. In a bowl, combine chopped spinach, quartered artichoke hearts, halved cherry tomatoes, and sliced Kalamata olives.
2. Toss with olive oil, lemon juice, minced garlic, salt, and pepper. Mix with cooked chickpea pasta.

Recipe 7. Sweet Potato and Lentil Curry

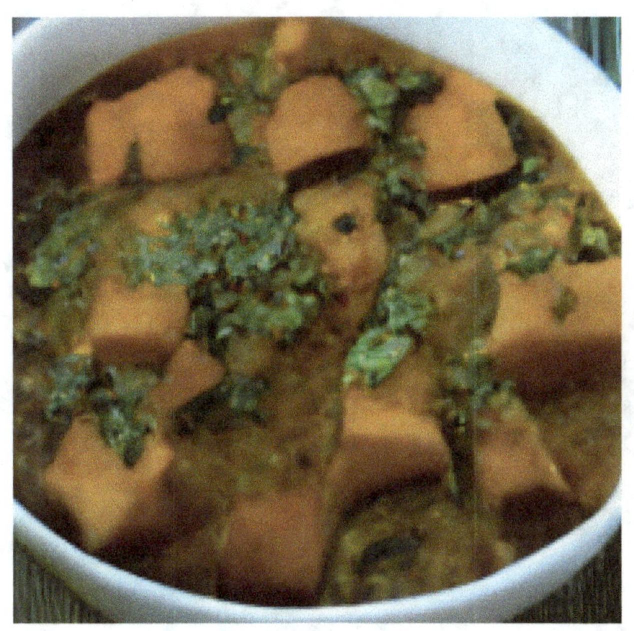

Ingredients:

- Red lentils, soaked
- Sweet potatoes, diced
- Coconut milk
- Onion, finely chopped
- Tomatoes, diced
- Curry powder, turmeric, cumin
- Garam masala
- Fresh cilantro, chopped
- Brown rice (optional for serving)

Preparation:

1. Sauté chopped onion until translucent. Add soaked red lentils, diced sweet potatoes, coconut milk, diced tomatoes, curry powder, turmeric, cumin, and garam masala.
2. Simmer until lentils and sweet potatoes are tender. Garnish with fresh cilantro. Serve over brown rice if desired.

Recipe 8. Black-Eyed Pea and Collard Greens Stew

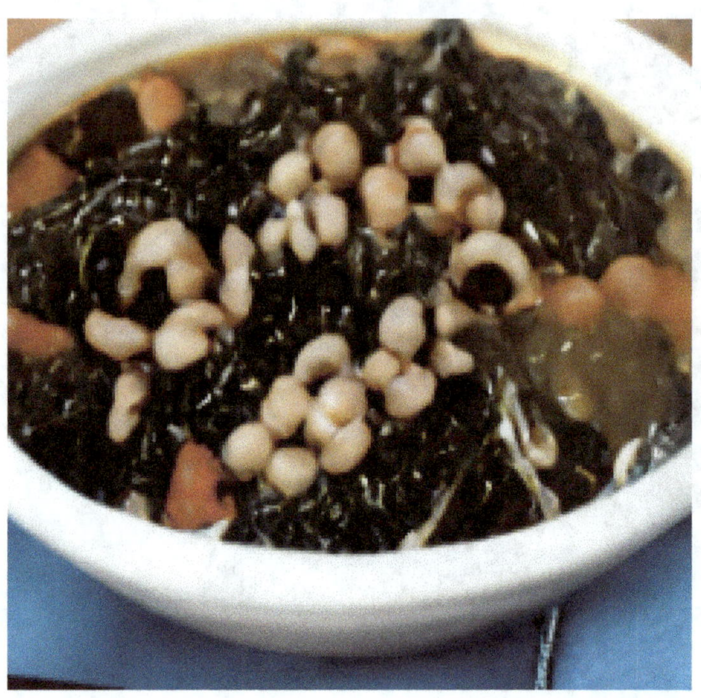

Ingredients:

- Black-eyed peas, soaked
- Collard greens, chopped
- Tomatoes, diced
- Onion, chopped
- Garlic, minced
- Vegetable broth
- Smoked paprika, cayenne pepper
- Apple cider vinegar
- Cornbread (optional for serving)

Preparation:

1. Sauté chopped onion and garlic until fragrant. Add soaked black-eyed peas, chopped collard greens, diced tomatoes, vegetable broth, smoked paprika, cayenne pepper, and apple cider vinegar.
2. Simmer until peas are tender. Serve with cornbread if desired.

Recipe 9. Eggplant and Chickpea Tagine

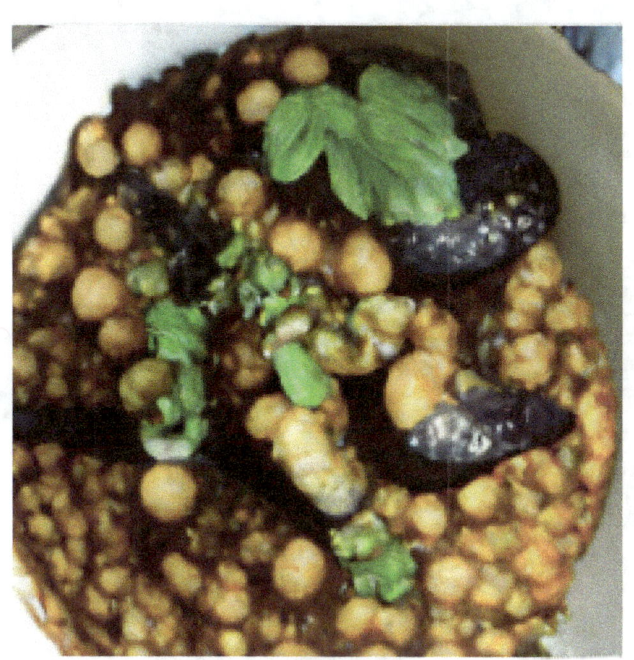

Ingredients:

- Eggplant, diced
- Chickpeas, cooked
- Tomatoes, diced
- Onion, finely chopped
- Apricots, dried and chopped
- Vegetable broth
- Ras el Hanout spice blend
- Couscous (optional for serving)

Preparation:

1. Sauté diced eggplant and finely chopped onion until softened. Add cooked chickpeas, diced tomatoes, dried apricots, vegetable broth, and Ras el Hanout spice blend.
2. Simmer until flavors meld. Serve over couscous if desired.

Recipe 10. Cauliflower and Lentil Shepherd's Pie

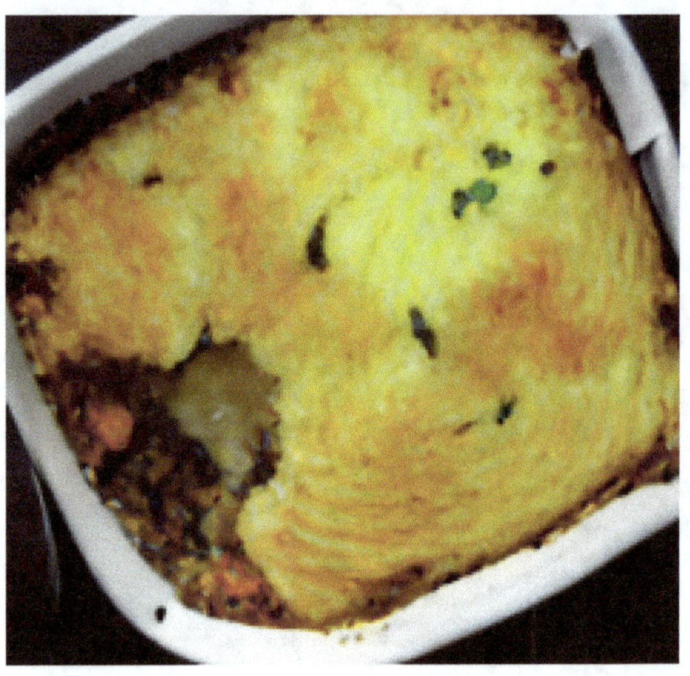

Ingredients:

- Lentils, cooked
- Cauliflower, mashed
- Carrots, diced
- Peas
- Onion, finely chopped
- Vegetable broth
- Tomato paste
- Rosemary, thyme
- Garlic, minced
- Mashed sweet potatoes (optional topping)

Preparation:

1. Sauté chopped onion and minced garlic until golden. Add cooked lentils, diced carrots, peas, vegetable broth, tomato paste, rosemary, and thyme.

2. Simmer until carrots are tender.

3. Layer in a baking dish and top with mashed cauliflower or sweet potatoes. Bake until the top is golden.

Flavorful Stir-Fries and Grain Bowls

Recipe 1. Teriyaki Vegetable Stir-Fry

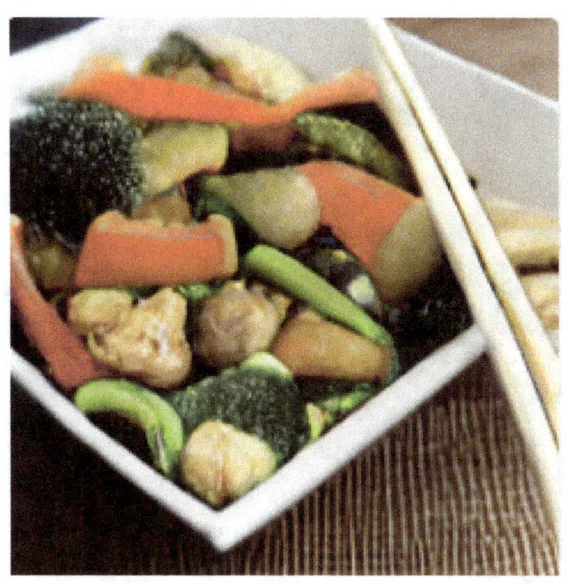

Ingredients:

- Broccoli florets
- Snap peas
- Carrots, julienned
- Bell peppers, sliced
- Tofu or tempeh cubed
- Teriyaki sauce
- Sesame oil
- Brown rice or quinoa (optional for serving)

Preparation:

1. Stir-fry broccoli, snap peas, julienned carrots, sliced bell peppers, and cubed tofu or tempeh in sesame oil.
2. Add teriyaki sauce and toss until vegetables are crisp-tender.
3. May be served atop brown rice or quinoa.

Recipe 2. Spicy Garlic Shrimp and Vegetable Stir-Fry

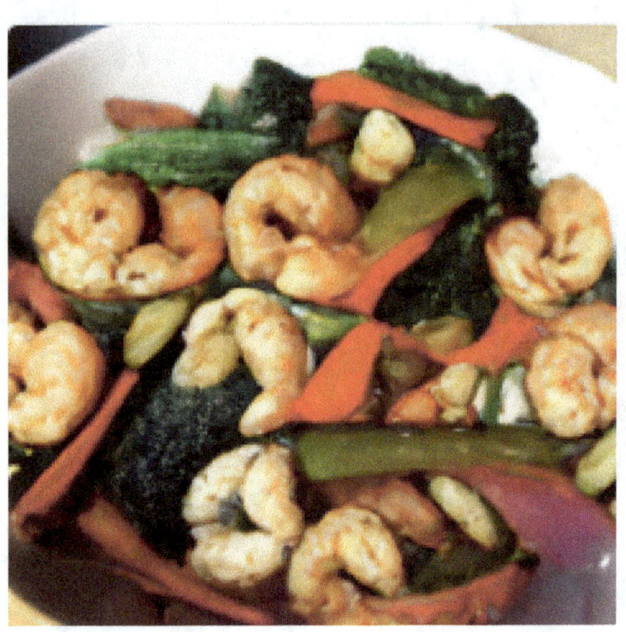

Ingredients:

- Shrimp, peeled and deveined
- Broccoli florets
- Bell peppers, sliced
- Snow peas
- Garlic, minced
- Red pepper flakes
- Soy sauce
- Rice noodles or jasmine rice (optional for serving)

Preparation:

1. Sauté shrimp, broccoli, bell peppers, snow peas, minced garlic, and red pepper flakes in a wok.
2. Add soy sauce and stir until shrimp are cooked. Serve over rice noodles or jasmine rice if desired.

Recipe 3. Mediterranean Chickpea and Couscous Bowl

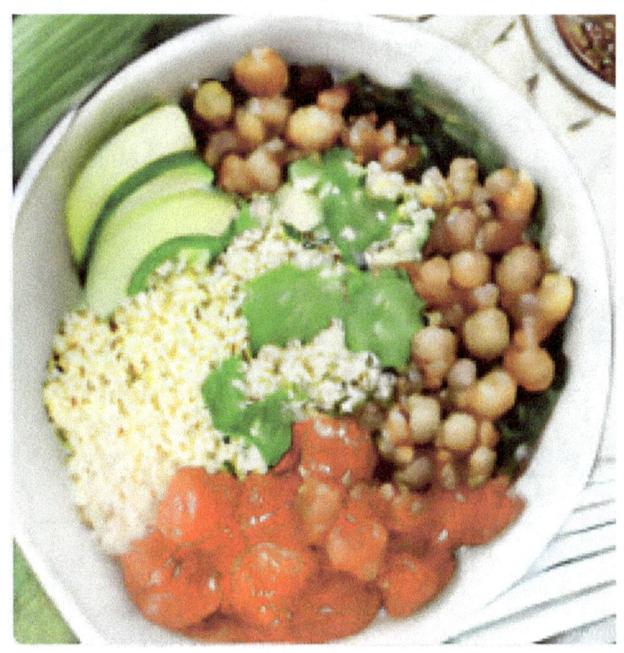

Ingredients:

- Chickpeas, cooked
- Cherry tomatoes, halved
- Cucumber, diced
- Kalamata olives, sliced
- Red onion, finely chopped
- Feta cheese, crumbled
- Lemon-tahini dressing
- Couscous

Preparation:

1. Combine cooked chickpeas with halved cherry tomatoes, diced cucumber, sliced Kalamata olives, finely chopped red onion, and crumbled feta cheese.
2. Drizzle with lemon-tahini dressing. Serve over couscous..

Recipe 4. Ginger Sesame Tofu and Vegetable Bowl

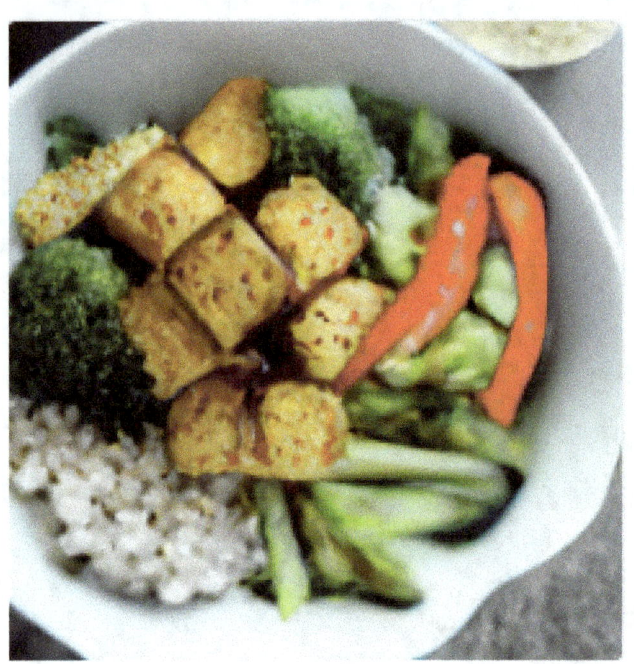

Ingredients:

- Tofu cubed
- Broccoli florets
- Carrots, julienned
- Bell peppers, sliced
- Green onions, sliced
- Ginger, minced
- Soy sauce
- Sesame seeds
- Brown rice or quinoa (optional for serving)

Preparation:

1. Sauté cubed tofu, broccoli, julienned carrots, sliced bell peppers, sliced green onions, and minced ginger in a wok.
2. Add soy sauce and toss until tofu is golden. Sprinkle with sesame seeds.
3. May be served atop brown rice or quinoa.

Recipe 5. Thai Basil Chicken and Vegetable Stir-Fry

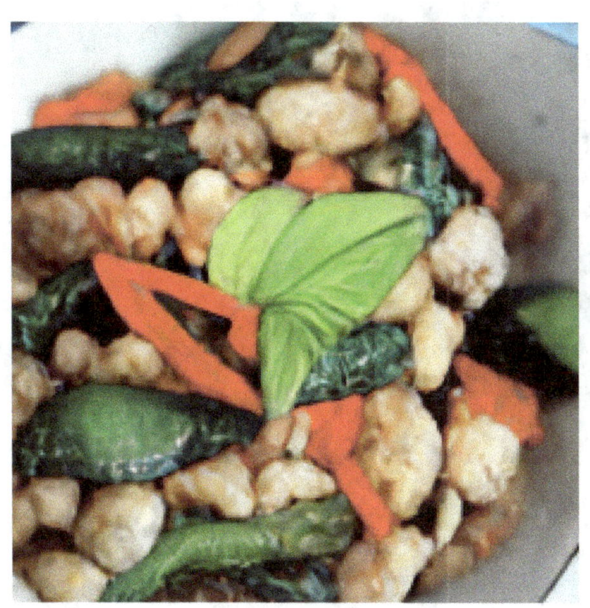

Ingredients:

- Chicken breast, thinly sliced
- Bell peppers, sliced
- Snap peas
- Carrots, julienned
- Thai basil leaves
- Garlic, minced
- Fish sauce or soy sauce
- Jasmine rice (optional for serving)

Preparation:

1. Stir-fried sliced chicken breast, bell peppers, snap peas, julienned carrots, minced garlic, and Thai basil leaves.
2. Add fish sauce or soy sauce and cook until chicken is done.
3. Serve over jasmine rice if desired.

Recipe 6. BBQ Jackfruit and Black Bean Burrito Bowl

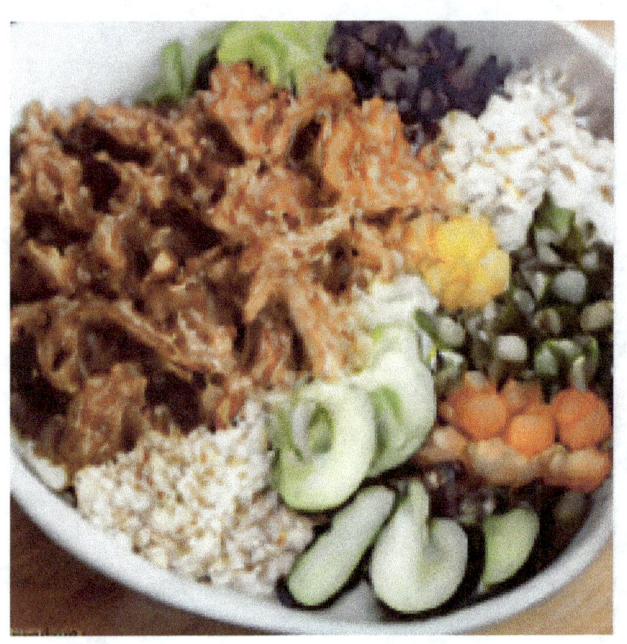

Ingredients:

- Jackfruit shredded
- Black beans, cooked
- Corn kernels, fresh or roasted
- Avocado, sliced
- Red cabbage shredded
- Lime wedges
- BBQ sauce
- Quinoa or brown rice (optional for serving)

Preparation:

1. Combine shredded jackfruit with cooked black beans, corn kernels, sliced avocado, shredded red cabbage, and lime wedges.
2. Drizzle with BBQ sauce. Serve over quinoa or brown rice if desired.

Recipe 7. Sesame Ginger Beef and Vegetable Stir-Fry

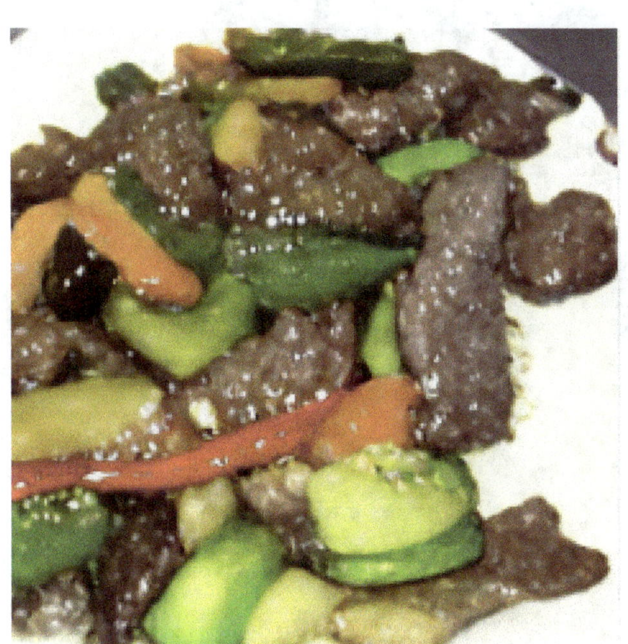

Ingredients:

- Beef strips
- Broccoli florets
- Bell peppers, sliced
- Snow peas
- Ginger, minced
- Soy sauce
- Sesame oil
- Rice noodles or jasmine rice (optional for serving)

Preparation:

1. Stir-fry beef strips, broccoli, sliced bell peppers, snow peas, and minced ginger in sesame oil.

2. Add soy sauce and toss until beef is cooked. Serve over rice noodles or jasmine rice if desired.

Recipe 8. Southwest Black Bean and Quinoa Bowl

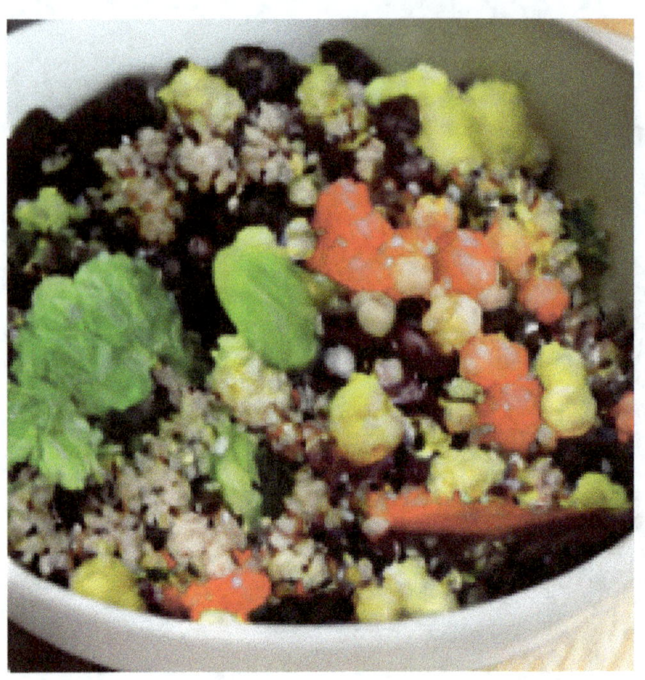

Ingredients:

- Black beans, cooked
- Quinoa, cooked
- Corn kernels, fresh or roasted
- Cherry tomatoes, halved
- Avocado, diced
- Cilantro, chopped
- Lime wedges
- Chipotle-lime dressing

Preparation:

1. Combine cooked black beans with cooked quinoa, fresh or roasted corn kernels, halved cherry tomatoes, diced avocado, chopped cilantro, and lime wedges.

2. Drizzle with chipotle-lime dressing..

Recipe 9. Pineapple Teriyaki Chicken and Vegetable Bowl

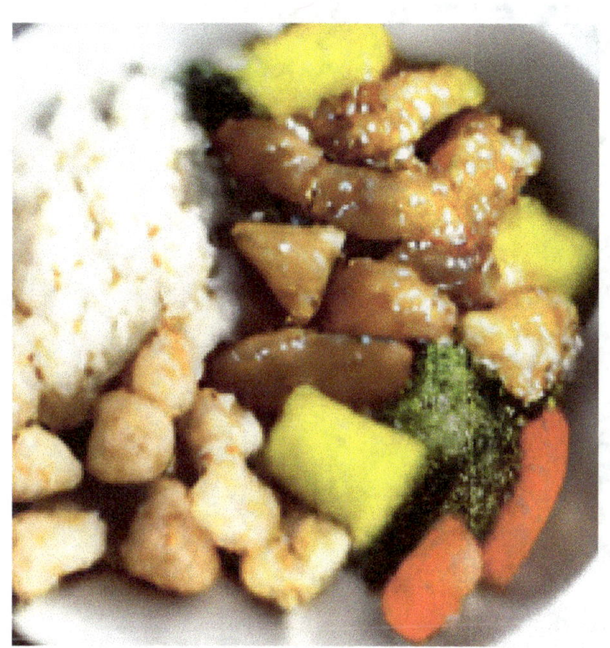

Ingredients:

- Chicken thighs, boneless and skinless, sliced
- Pineapple chunks
- Bell peppers, sliced
- Red onion, sliced
- Snow peas
- Teriyaki sauce
- Brown rice or quinoa (optional for serving)

Preparation:

1. Sauté sliced chicken thighs, pineapple chunks, sliced bell peppers, sliced red onion, and snow peas in a wok.

2. Add teriyaki sauce and toss until the chicken is cooked. May be served atop brown rice or quinoa.

Recipe 10. Lemon Garlic Shrimp and Asparagus Quinoa Bowl

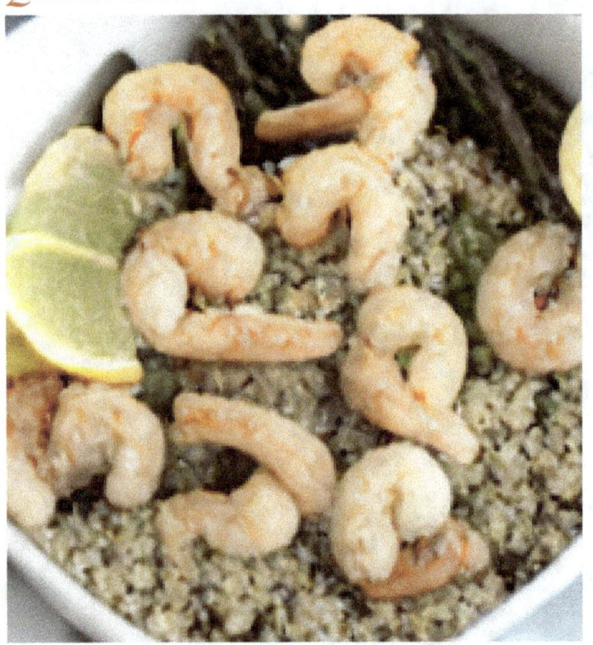

Ingredients:

- Shrimp, peeled and deveined
- Asparagus spears, trimmed
- Lemon zest and juice
- Garlic, minced
- Quinoa, cooked
- Fresh parsley, chopped
- Olive oil
- Salt and pepper to taste

Preparation:

1. Sauté shrimp and trimmed asparagus spears in olive oil with lemon zest and minced garlic.
2. Add lemon juice and cook until shrimp are pink and asparagus is tender.
3. Serve over cooked quinoa. Garnish with chopped fresh parsley.

Flavorful Stir-Fries and Grain Bowls

Recipe 1. Classic Baked Ziti with Vegan Ricotta

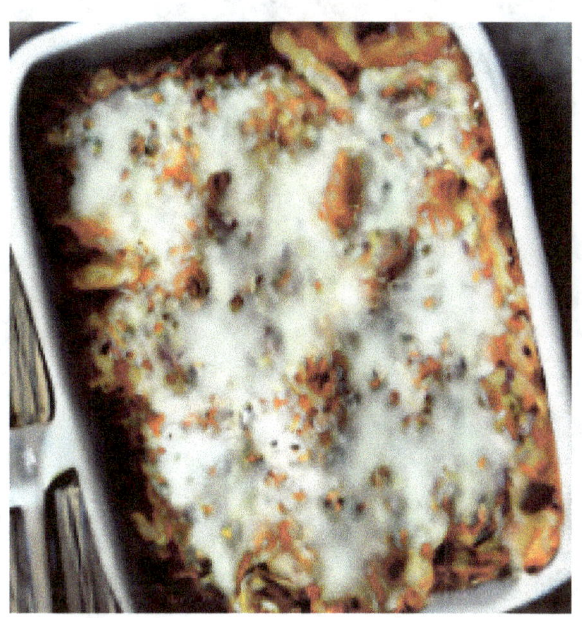

Ingredients:

- Ziti pasta, cooked
- Marinara sauce
- Vegan ricotta cheese
- Vegan mozzarella, shredded
- Fresh basil, chopped
- Garlic powder, onion powder
- Salt and pepper to taste

Preparation:

1. Mix cooked ziti pasta with marinara sauce, vegan ricotta cheese, and vegan mozzarella.
2. Season liberally with a blend of garlic powder, onion powder, salt, and pepper.
3. Bake until bubbling. Garnish with fresh basil before serving.

Recipe 2. Creamy Spinach and Artichoke Baked Dip

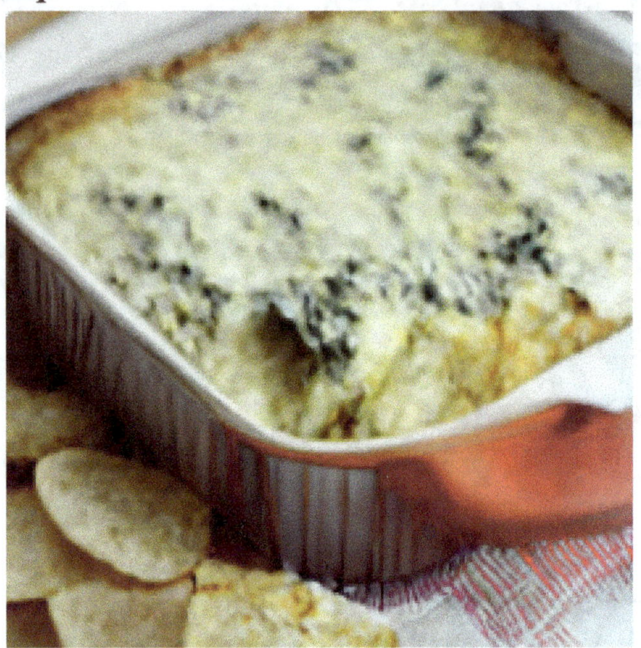

Ingredients:

- Spinach, chopped
- Artichoke hearts, chopped
- Cream cheese (dairy or vegan)
- Sour cream or dairy-free alternative
- Garlic, minced
- Parmesan or vegan cheese, grated
- Bread or tortilla chips for dipping

Preparation:

1. Combine chopped spinach, chopped artichoke hearts, cream cheese, sour cream, minced garlic, and grated
2. Parmesan or vegan cheese. Bake until bubbly and golden.
3. Serve with bread or tortilla chips for dipping.

Recipe 3. Shepherd's Pie with Mashed Cauliflower Topping

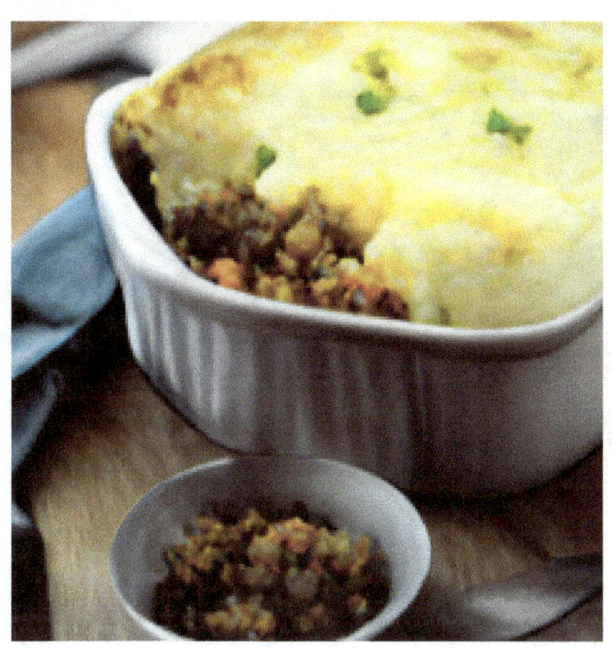

Ingredients:

- Lentils, cooked
- Mixed vegetables (peas, carrots, corn)
- Onion, chopped
- Tomato paste
- Vegetable broth
- Mashed cauliflower (as topping)
- Rosemary, thyme
- Salt and pepper to taste

Preparation:

1. Sauté chopped onion until translucent. Add cooked lentils, mixed vegetables, tomato paste, and vegetable broth.
2. Simmer until vegetables are tender.
3. Transfer to a baking dish. Top with mashed cauliflower.
4. Bake until the topping is golden. Infuse with rosemary, thyme, and a touch of salt and pepper.

Recipe 4. Baked Eggplant Parmesan

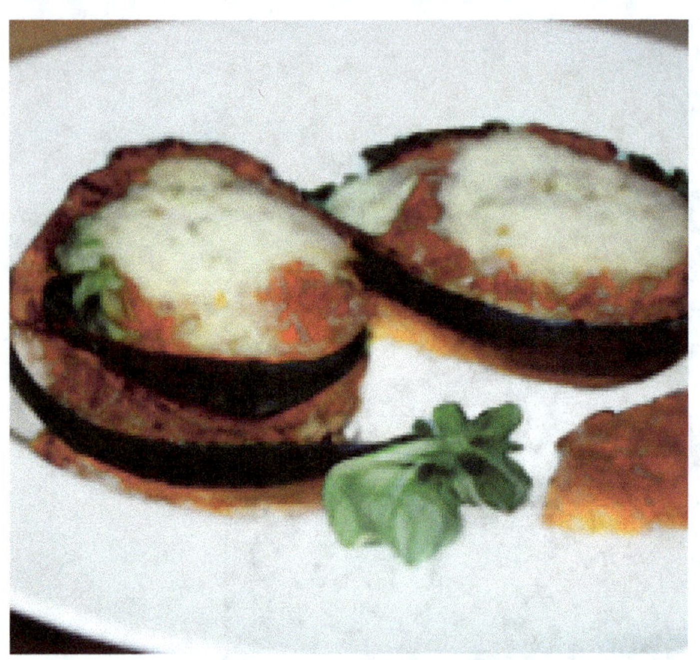

Ingredients:

- Eggplant, sliced
- Bread crumbs (regular or panko)
- Marinara sauce
- Mozzarella cheese, shredded
- Parmesan cheese, grated
- Fresh basil, chopped
- Olive oil
- Salt and pepper to taste

Preparation:

1. Dip eggplant slices in olive oil and coat with bread crumbs. Bake until golden.
2. In a baking dish, layer baked eggplant slices with marinara sauce, shredded mozzarella, and grated Parmesan.
3. Repeat layers.
4. Bake until bubbly. Garnish with chopped fresh basil..

Recipe 5. Cheesy Broccoli and Rice Casserole

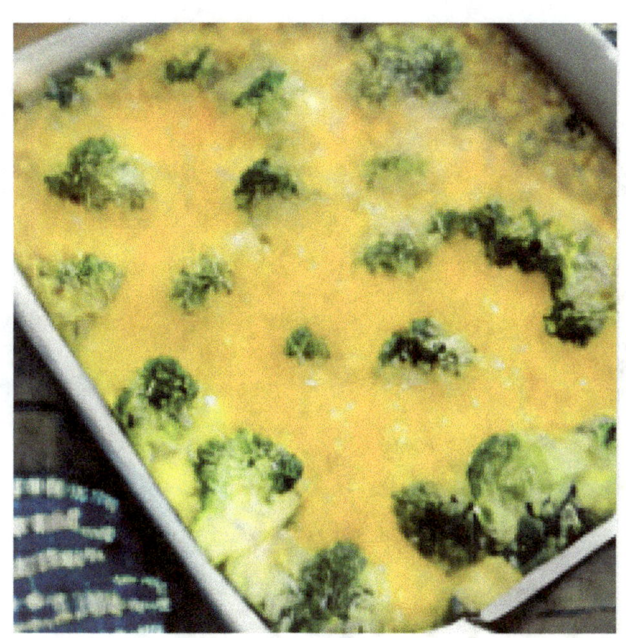

Ingredients:

- Broccoli florets, steamed
- Cooked brown rice
- Cheddar cheese, shredded
- Sour cream or Greek yogurt
- Onion, finely chopped
- Garlic powder, onion powder
- Salt and pepper to taste

Preparation:

1. Combine steamed broccoli florets, cooked brown rice, shredded cheddar cheese, sour cream or Greek yogurt, finely chopped onion, garlic powder, onion powder, salt, and pepper.
2. Transfer to a baking dish. Bake until the cheese is fully melted and exhibiting visible signs of bubbling

Recipe 6. Stuffed Bell Peppers with Quinoa and Black Beans

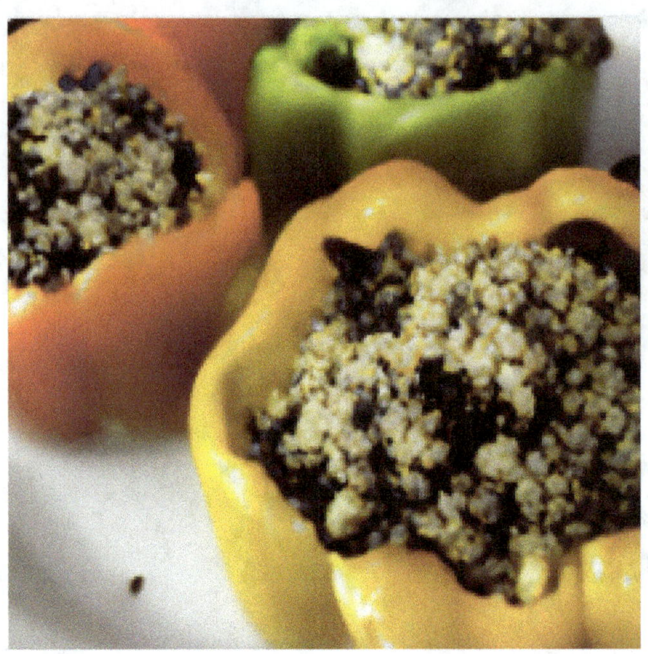

Ingredients:

- Bell peppers, halved
- Quinoa, cooked
- Black beans, cooked
- Corn kernels, fresh or roasted
- Salsa
- Cumin, chili powder
- Vegan cheese (optional)
- Avocado, sliced (for garnish)

Preparation:

1. Combine cooked quinoa with black beans, fresh or roasted corn kernels, salsa, cumin, and chili powder.
2. Stuff halved bell peppers with the quinoa mixture. Optional: Sprinkle with vegan cheese.
3. Bake until the peppers are tender.
4. Garnish with sliced avocado.

Recipe 7. Baked Macaroni and Cheese

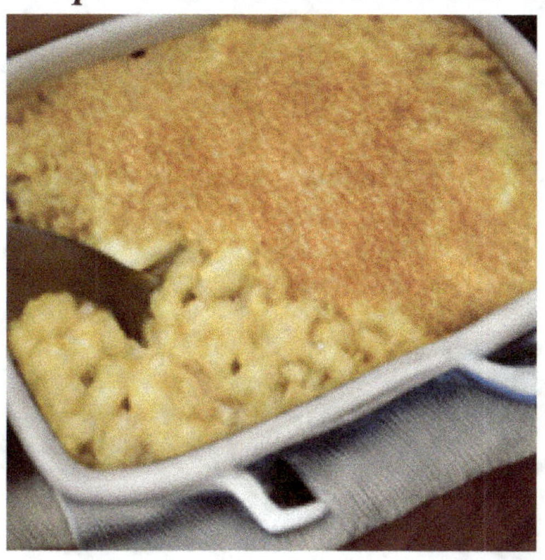

Ingredients:

- Elbow macaroni, cooked
- Cheddar cheese, shredded
- Milk or plant-based milk
- Butter or vegan butter
- All-purpose flour
- Mustard powder
- Salt and pepper to taste

Preparation:

1. Cook elbow macaroni according to package instructions.
2. Heat butter in a saucepan until liquified, then incorporate flour by whisking to form a roux. Add milk and continue whisking until thickened.
3. Stir in shredded cheddar cheese until melted. Season with mustard powder, salt, and pepper.
4. Combine with cooked macaroni.
5. Transfer to a baking dish.
6. Bake until golden and bubbly.

Recipe 8. Sweet Potato and Black Bean Enchilada Casserole

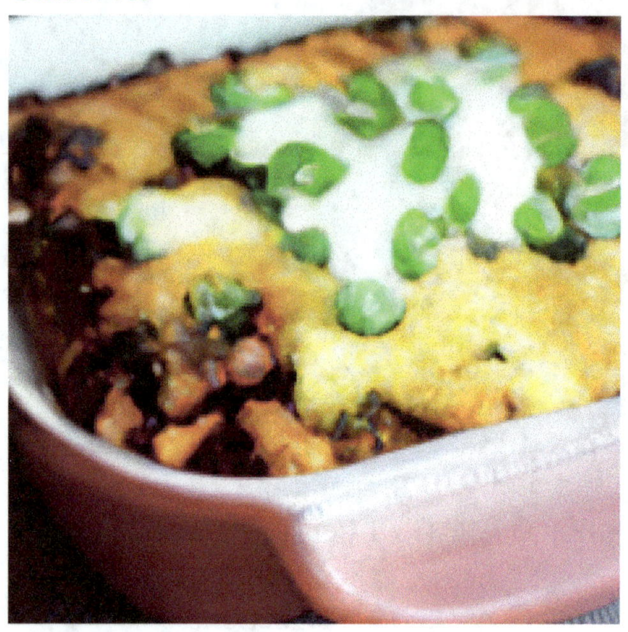

Ingredients:

- Sweet potatoes, diced and roasted
- Black beans, cooked
- Corn tortillas
- Enchilada sauce
- Vegan cheese, shredded
- Avocado, sliced
- Cilantro chopped (for garnish)

Preparation:

1. Layer roasted sweet potatoes, cooked black beans, and corn tortillas in a baking dish.
2. Pour enchilada sauce over each layer and sprinkle with shredded vegan cheese.
3. Repeat layers. Bake until bubbly.
4. Finished with slivered avocado and a sprinkle of cilantro.

Recipe 9. Mediterranean Quinoa and Vegetable Bake

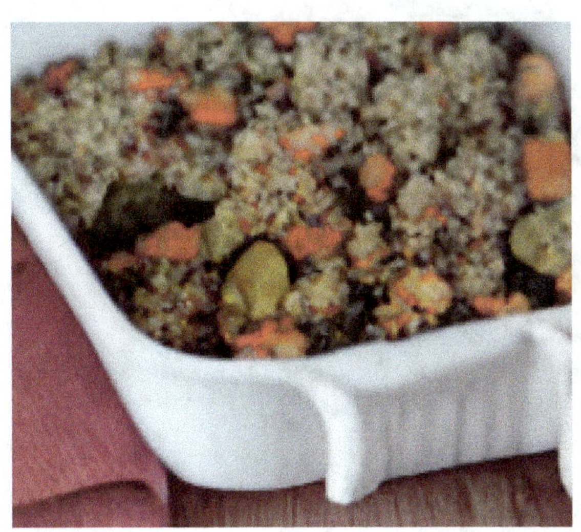

Ingredients:

- Quinoa, cooked
- Cherry tomatoes, halved
- Kalamata olives, sliced
- Artichoke hearts, quartered
- Red onion, thinly sliced
- Feta cheese, crumbled
- Olive oil
- Lemon juice
- Oregano, thyme
- Salt and pepper to taste

Preparation:

1. Mix cooked quinoa with halved cherry tomatoes, sliced Kalamata olives, quartered artichoke hearts, thinly sliced red onion, and crumbled feta cheese.

2. Drizzle with olive oil and lemon juice. Season with oregano, thyme, salt, and pepper.

3. Transfer to a baking dish. Bake until heated through.

Recipe 10. Teriyaki Tofu and Vegetable Casserole

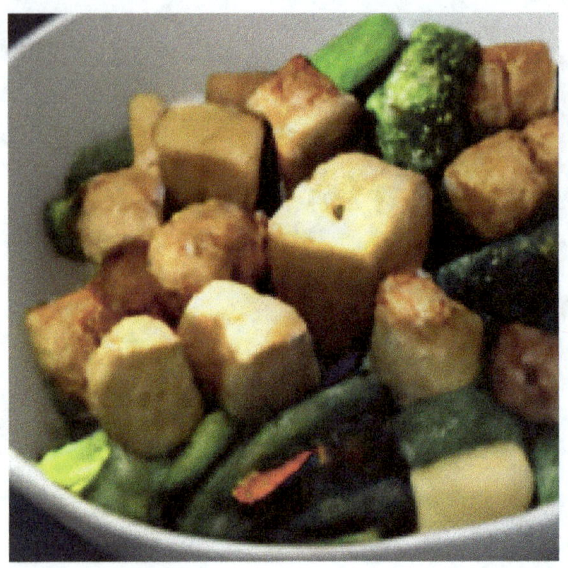

Ingredients:

- Tofu cubed
- Broccoli florets
- Carrots, sliced
- Snap peas
- Teriyaki sauce
- Brown rice or quinoa (optional for serving)

Preparation:

1. Sauté cubed tofu, broccoli florets, sliced carrots, and snap peas in teriyaki sauce.
2. Transfer to a baking dish. Bake until tofu is golden and vegetables are tender.
3. May be enjoyed atop brown rice or quinoa.

Chapter 6
Snacks and Appetizers
Guilt-Free Snacking with Plant-Based Options

Recipe 1. Crunchy Kale Chips

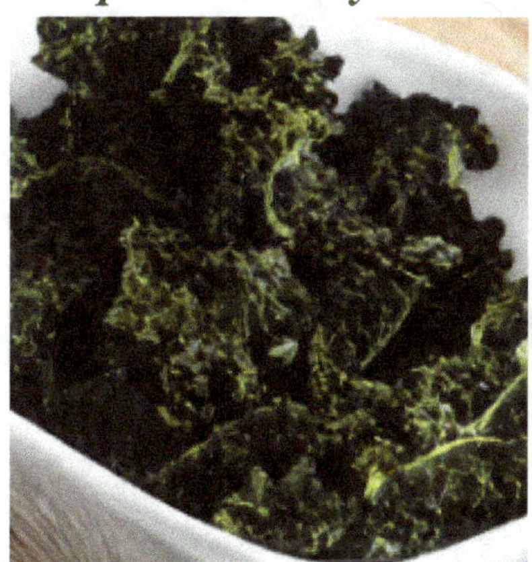

Ingredients:

- Fresh kale leaves, washed and dried
- Olive oil
- Nutritional yeast
- Garlic powder
- Salt and pepper to taste

Preparation:

1. Preheat the oven to 350°F (175°C).
2. Tear kale leaves into bite-sized pieces, removing the tough stems.
3. Toss kale with olive oil, nutritional yeast, garlic powder, salt, and pepper.
4. Spread the kale on a baking sheet in a single layer.
5. Bake for 10-15 minutes, or until the edges are crisp but not burnt.
6. Allow to cool before serving.

Recipe 2. Smoky Roasted Chickpeas

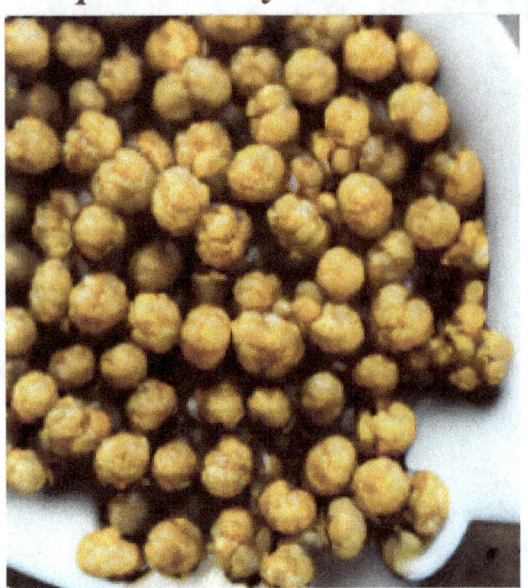

Ingredients:

- Chickpeas, cooked and drained
- Smoked paprika
- Cumin
- Garlic powder
- Olive oil
- Salt and cayenne pepper to taste

Preparation:

1. Preheat the oven to 400°F (200°C).
2. In a bowl, toss chickpeas with smoked paprika, cumin, garlic powder, olive oil, salt, and cayenne pepper.
3. Arrange the chickpeas evenly across a baking sheet, ensuring no overlap.
4. Roast for 25-30 minutes, shaking the pan occasionally, until the chickpeas are golden and crunchy.
5. Cool before serving.

Recipe 3. Stuffed Mini Bell Peppers

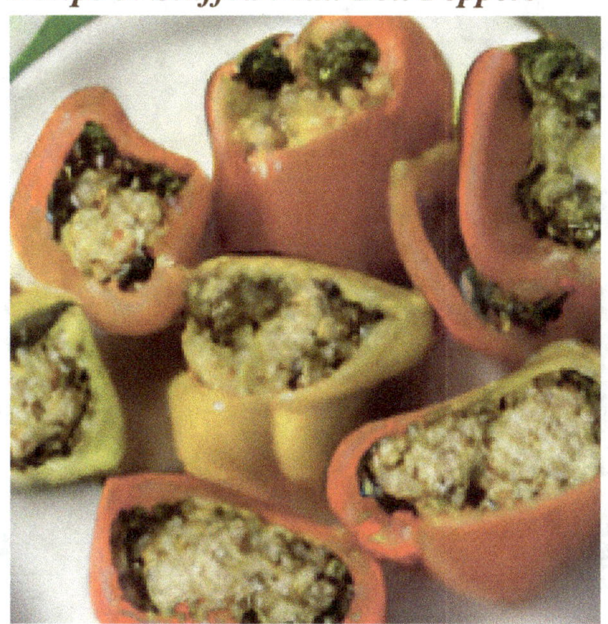

Ingredients:

- Mini bell peppers, halved and seeds removed
- Hummus
- Cherry tomatoes, quartered
- Cucumber, diced
- Fresh parsley, chopped
- Lemon zest
- Salt and pepper to taste

Preparation:

1. Fill each mini bell pepper half with a spoonful of hummus.
2. Top with quartered cherry tomatoes, diced cucumber, chopped fresh parsley, and a sprinkle of lemon zest.
3. Season with salt and pepper.
4. Arrange on a serving platter and enjoy.

Recipe 4. Spicy Edamame Pods

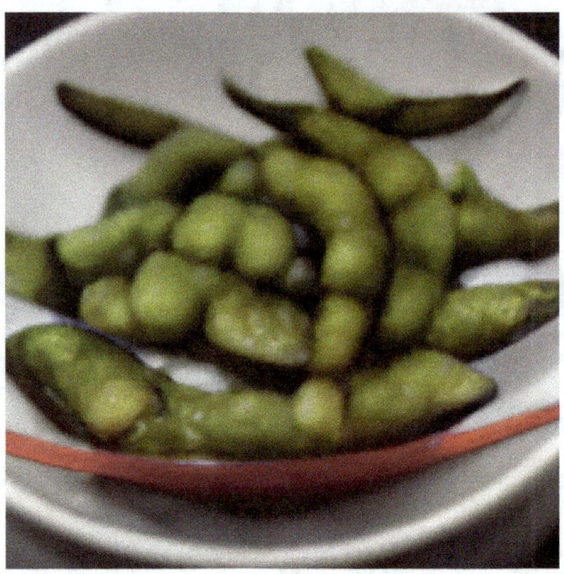

Ingredients:

- Edamame pods, thawed if frozen
- Sesame oil
- Soy sauce
- Sriracha sauce
- Sesame seeds
- Green onions, sliced

Preparation:

1. Steam or boil edamame pods until tender.
2. In a bowl, toss the edamame with sesame oil, soy sauce, and sriracha sauce to taste.
3. Garnish with toasted sesame seeds and julienned scallions.
4. Serve warm or at room temperature.

Recipe 5. Avocado and Black Bean Salsa

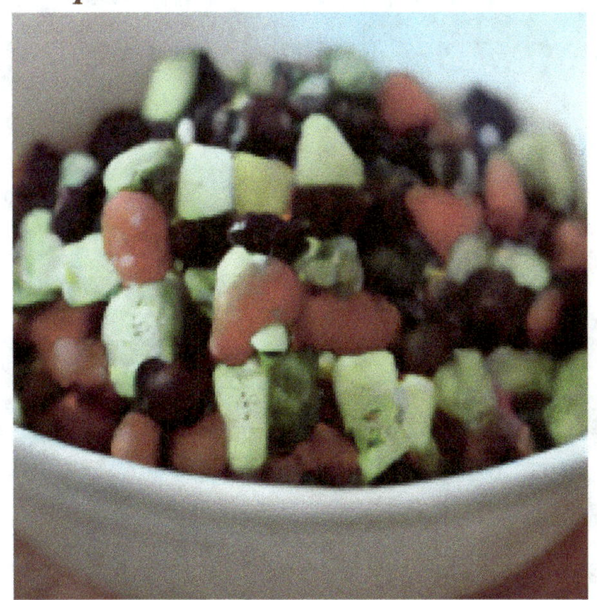

Ingredients:

- Avocado, diced
- Black beans, cooked and drained
- Corn kernels, fresh or roasted
- Red onion, finely chopped
- Cherry tomatoes, diced
- Cilantro, chopped
- Lime juice
- Salt and pepper to taste

Preparation:

1. In a bowl, combine diced avocado, black beans, corn kernels, finely chopped red onion, diced cherry tomatoes, and chopped cilantro.
2. Drizzle with lime juice and gently toss.
3. Season with salt and pepper.
4. Serve with tortilla chips or as a topping for whole-grain crackers.

119

Creative Vegetable Dips and Spreads

Recipe 1. Roasted Red Pepper and Walnut Dip

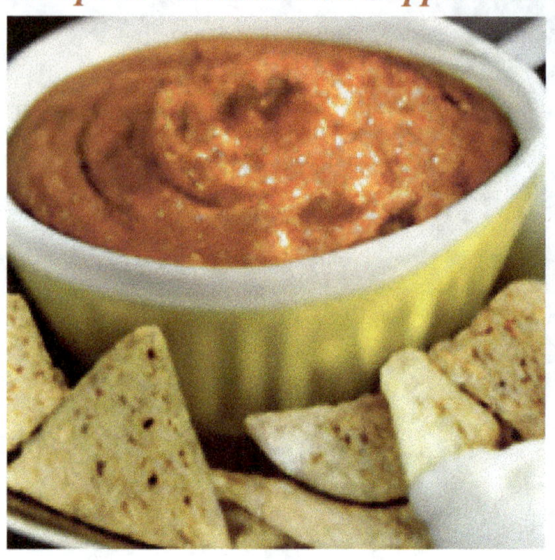

Ingredients:

- Roasted red peppers, peeled and seeded
- Walnuts, toasted
- Garlic, minced
- Lemon juice
- Olive oil
- Smoked paprika
- Salt and pepper to taste

Preparation:

1. In a food processor, combine roasted red peppers, toasted walnuts, minced garlic, and lemon juice.
2. Pulse until ingredients are finely chopped.
3. Drizzle in olive oil while continuing to blend until smooth.
4. Season with smoked paprika, salt, and pepper.
5. Serve as a dip with fresh vegetable crudites or pita bread.

Recipe 2. Caramelized Onion and White Bean Dip

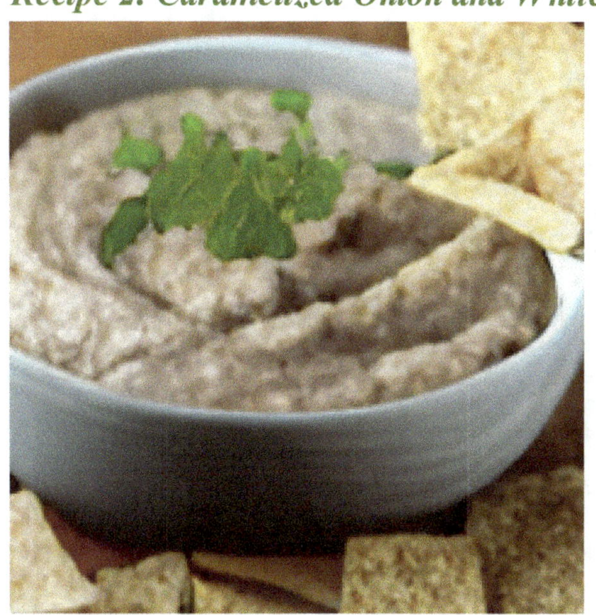

Ingredients:

- Roasted red peppers, Caramelized onions
- White beans, drained and rinsed
- Greek yogurt or plant-based yogurt
- Dijon mustard
- Fresh thyme leaves
- Lemon zest
- Salt and pepper to taste

Preparation:

1. In a blender, combine caramelized onions, white beans, Greek yogurt or plant-based yogurt, and Dijon mustard.
2. Blend until smooth and creamy.
3. Stir in fresh thyme leaves and lemon zest.
4. Season with salt and pepper.
5. Serve as a spread on whole grain crackers or as a dip for vegetable sticks.

Recipe 3. Spicy Avocado and Black Bean Hummus

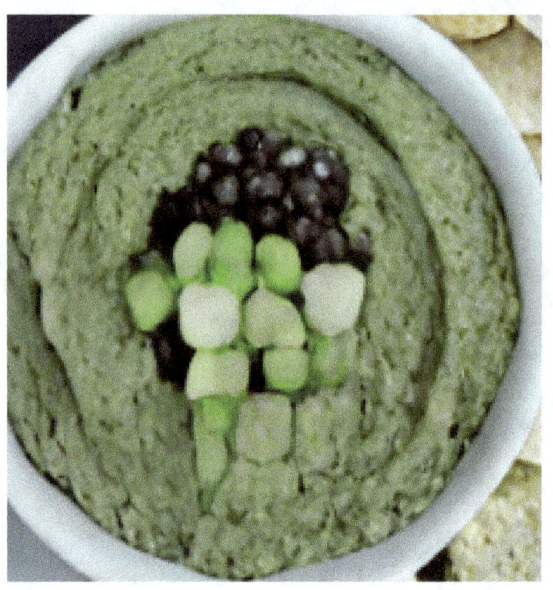

Ingredients:

- Avocado, peeled and pitted
- Black beans, cooked and drained
- Chickpeas, cooked and drained
- Jalapeño, seeded and chopped
- Cilantro, chopped
- Lime juice
- Cumin
- Salt and pepper to taste

Preparation:

1. In a food processor, combine avocado, black beans, chickpeas, chopped jalapeño, and cilantro.
2. Blend until smooth.
3. Add lime juice and cumin; blend until well combined.
4. Season with salt and pepper.
5. Serve as a spicy hummus dip with tortilla chips or vegetable slices.

Recipe 4. Sun-Dried Tomato and Basil Pesto

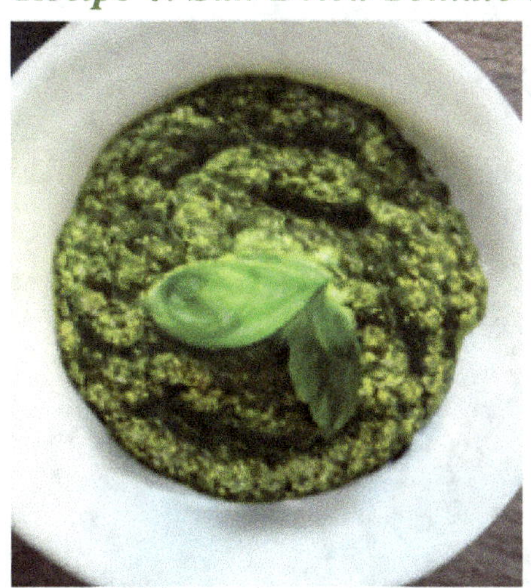

Ingredients:

- Sun-dried tomatoes, soaked in hot water
- Fresh basil leaves
- Pine nuts, toasted
- Garlic, minced
- Nutritional yeast
- Olive oil
- Lemon juice
- Salt and pepper to taste

Preparation:

1. Drain soaked sun-dried tomatoes and place them in a food processor.
2. Add fresh basil leaves, toasted pine nuts, minced garlic, and nutritional yeast.
3. Pulse until coarsely chopped.
4. With the processor running, drizzle in olive oil and lemon juice until desired consistency is reached.
5. Season with salt and pepper.
6. Use as a flavorful spread on sandwiches or as a dip for veggie platters.

Recipe 5. Curry-Spiced Carrot and Cashew Dip

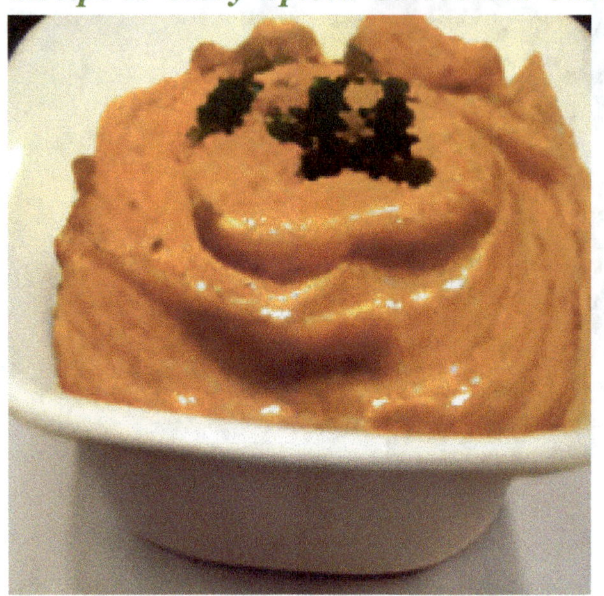

Ingredients:

- Carrots, peeled and chopped
- Cashews, roasted
- Coconut milk
- Curry powder
- Ginger, grated
- Maple syrup or agave nectar
- Cilantro, chopped
- Salt and pepper to taste

Preparation:

1. Steam or boil carrots until tender; let them cool.
2. In a blender, combine cooked carrots, roasted cashews, coconut milk, curry powder, grated ginger, and maple syrup or agave nectar.
3. Blend until smooth.
4. Incorporate the cilantro and adjust the seasoning with salt and pepper.
5. Serve as a dip with carrot sticks or as a spread on whole grain bread.

Quick and Easy Energy Bites

Recipe 1. Almond Joy Energy Bites

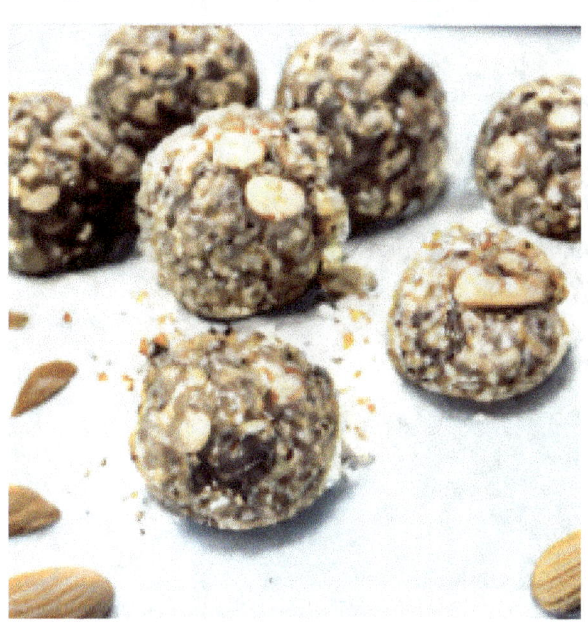

Ingredients:

- Almonds, raw
- Dates, pitted
- Shredded coconut
- Cocoa powder
- Vanilla extract
- Pinch of salt

Preparation:

1. In a food processor, blend raw almonds until finely chopped.
2. Add pitted dates, shredded coconut, cocoa powder, vanilla extract, and a pinch of salt.
3. Blend until the mixture sticks together.
4. Roll into bite-sized balls.
5. Refrigerate for at least 30 minutes before enjoying.

Recipe 2. Peanut Butter Banana Oat Bites

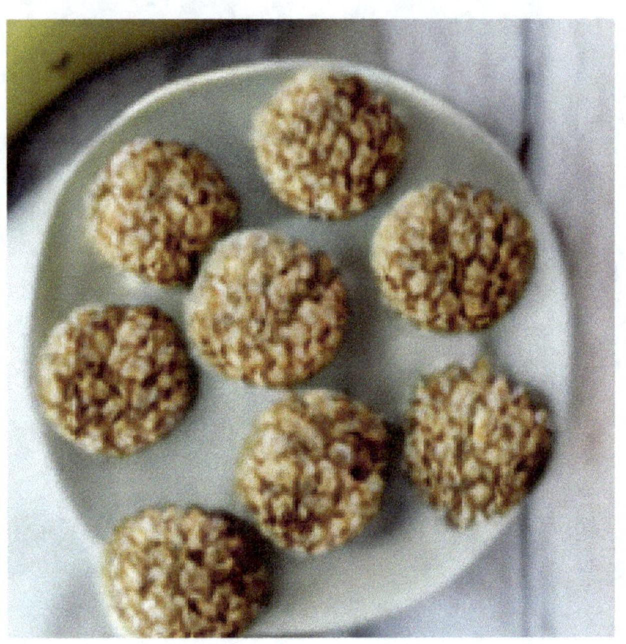

Ingredients:

- Rolled oats
- Ripe bananas, mashed
- Peanut butter
- Honey or maple syrup
- Chia seeds
- Cinnamon

Preparation:

1. In a bowl, combine rolled oats, mashed bananas, peanut butter, honey or maple syrup, chia seeds, and a dash of cinnamon.
2. Mix until well combined.
3. Scoop out small portions and roll into bites.
4. Place in the freezer for 20-30 minutes to set.

Recipe 3. Berry Bliss Energy Bites

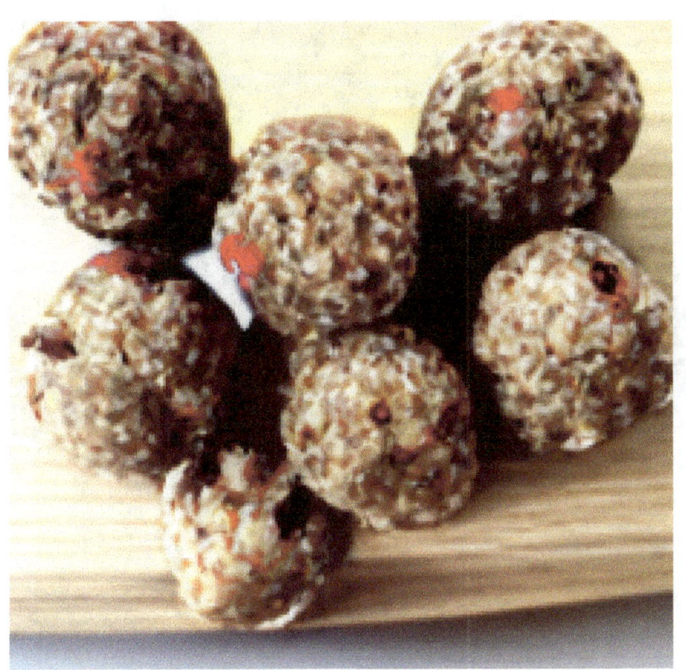

Ingredients:

- Mixed berries (strawberries, blueberries, raspberries)
- Almond flour
- Chia seeds
- Honey or agave nectar
- Rolled oats
- Coconut flakes

Preparation:

1. In a blender, pulse mixed berries until slightly chunky.
2. Transfer to a bowl and add almond flour, chia seeds, honey or agave nectar, rolled oats, and coconut flakes.
3. Mix thoroughly.
4. Form the mixture into bite-sized balls.
5. Chill in the refrigerator before serving.

Recipe 4. Chocolate Mint Protein Bites

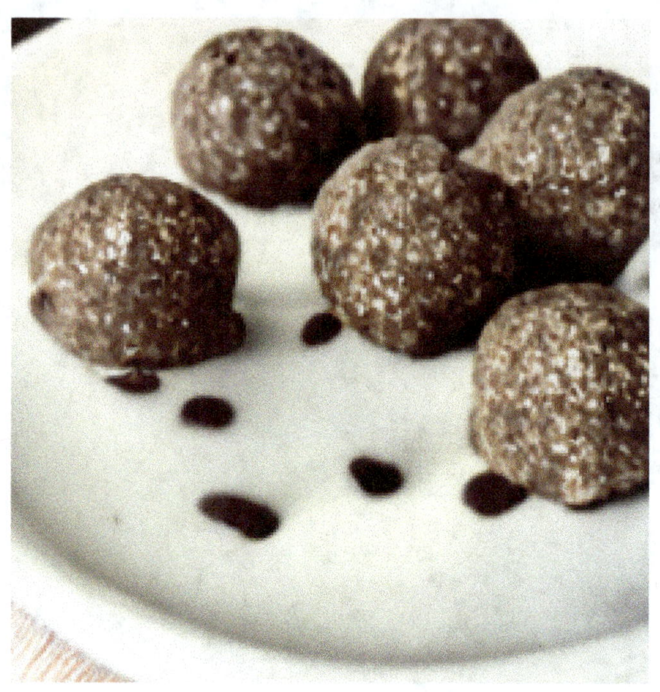

Ingredients:

- Chocolate protein powder
- Almond butter
- Medjool dates, pitted
- Peppermint extract
- Dark chocolate chips

Preparation:

1. In a food processor, combine chocolate protein powder, almond butter, pitted Medjool dates, and a few drops of peppermint extract.
2. Blend until a dough-like consistency is achieved.
3. Fold in dark chocolate chips.
4. Shape into small bites and refrigerate until firm.

Recipe 5. Tropical Paradise Energy Bites

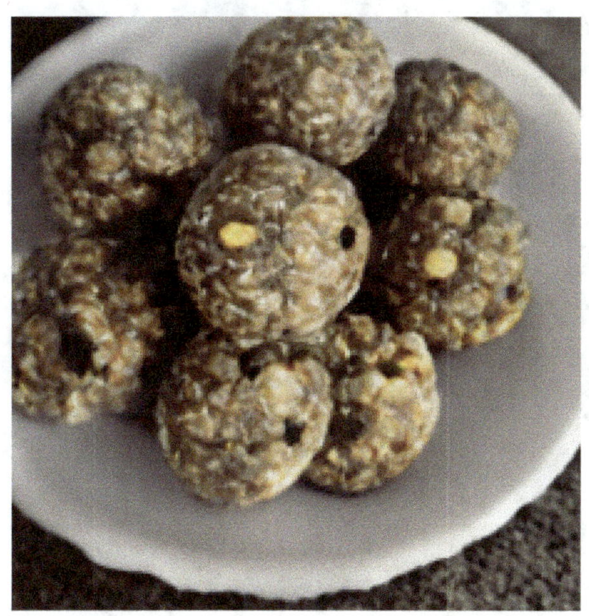

Ingredients:

- Dried pineapple, chopped
- Cashews
- Coconut oil
- Flaxseeds
- Vanilla extract
- Turmeric powder (optional for color)

Preparation:

1. In a food processor, blend dried pineapple and cashews until finely chopped.
2. Add coconut oil, flaxseeds, vanilla extract, and turmeric powder (optional).
3. Blend until the mixture forms a sticky dough.
4. Roll into bite-sized balls and refrigerate.

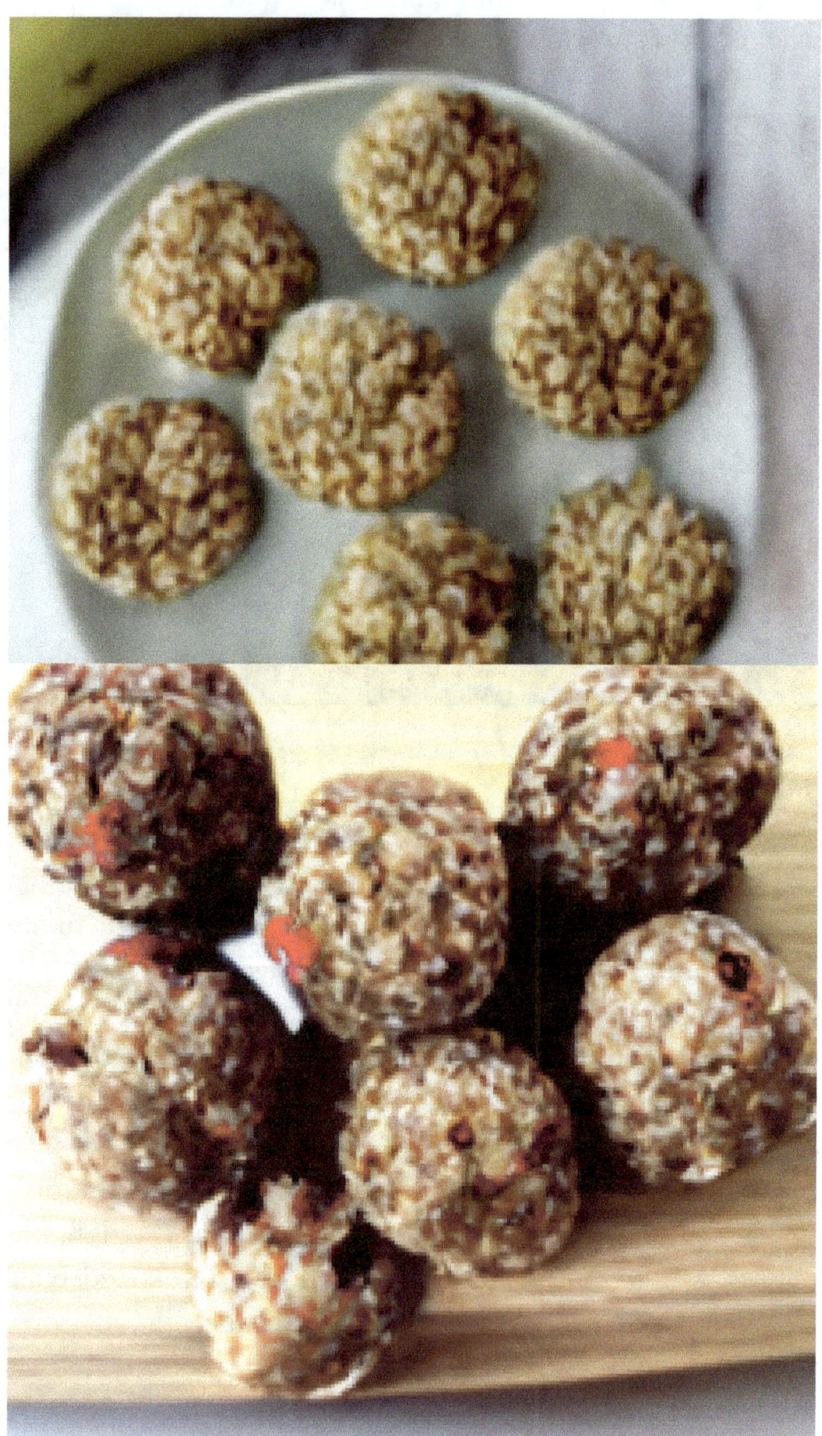

Chapter 7
Sweet Treats with a Purpose
Guilt-Free Snacking with Plant-Based Options

Recipe 1. Dark Chocolate Avocado Mousse

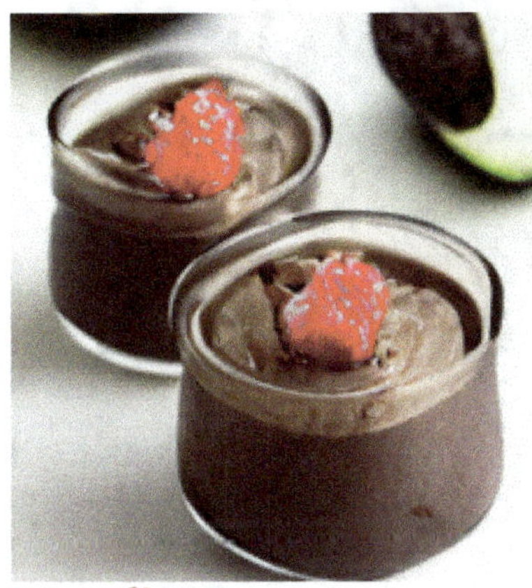

Ingredients:

- Ripe avocados
- Dark chocolate, melted
- Maple syrup or agave nectar
- Cocoa powder
- Vanilla extract
- Pinch of sea salt

Preparation:

1. In a blender, combine ripe avocados, melted dark chocolate, maple syrup or agave nectar, cocoa powder, vanilla extract, and a pinch of sea salt.
2. Blend until smooth and creamy.
3. Spoon into individual serving glasses.
4. Incorporate the cilantro and adjust the seasoning with salt and pepper.

Recipe 2. Berry-Infused Chia Seed Pudding

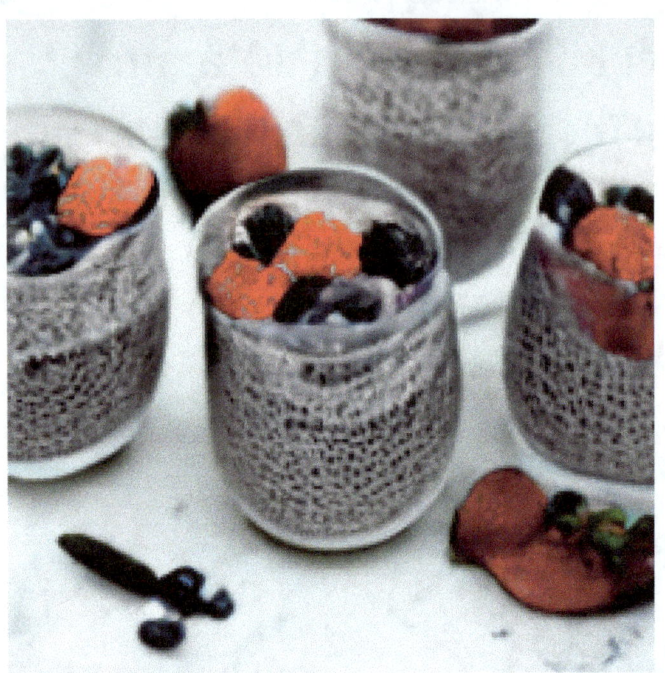

Ingredients:

- Mixed berries (blueberries, raspberries, strawberries)
- Chia seeds
- Almond milk or coconut milk
- Maple syrup or honey
- Vanilla extract

Preparation:

1. In a bowl, mash mixed berries with a fork.
2. Add chia seeds, almond milk or coconut milk, maple syrup or honey, and vanilla extract.
3. Stir well and let it sit in the refrigerator for at least four hours or overnight.
4. Serve chilled, topped with additional berries.

Recipe 3. Pomegranate and Pistachio Yogurt Parfait

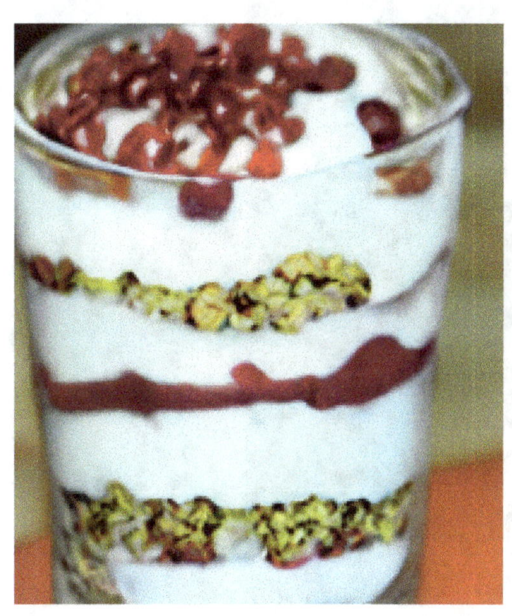

Ingredients:

- Greek yogurt or plant-based yogurt
- Pomegranate seeds
- Pistachios, chopped
- Honey or agave nectar
- Cinnamon

Preparation:

1. In a glass or bowl, layer Greek yogurt or plant-based yogurt with pomegranate seeds and chopped pistachios.
2. Drizzle with honey or agave nectar.
3. Sprinkle a dash of cinnamon on top.
4. Repeat the layers.
5. Garnish with additional pomegranate seeds and pistachios.

Recipe 4. Acai Berry Coconut Bliss Balls

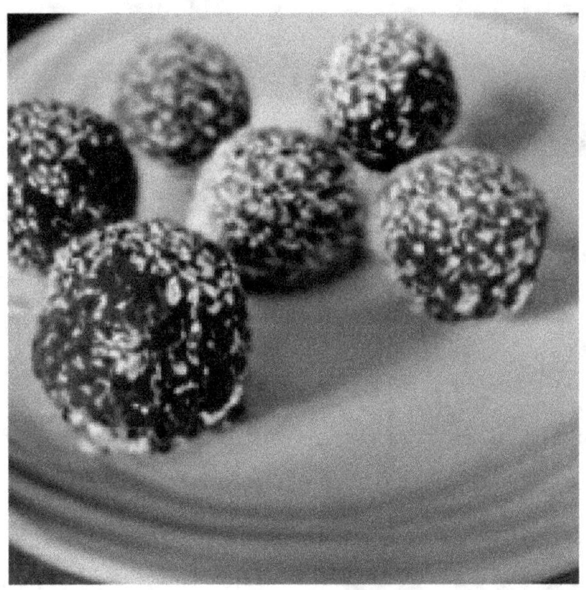

Ingredients:

- Acai berry powder
- Medjool dates, pitted
- Almond flour
- Shredded coconut
- Almond butter
- Vanilla extract

Preparation:

1. In a food processor, blend acai berry powder, pitted Medjool dates, almond flour, shredded coconut, almond butter, and vanilla extract until a sticky dough forms.
2. Roll the mixture into bite-sized balls.
3. Coat the balls with additional shredded coconut.
4. Gently incorporate the cilantro and adjust the seasoning with salt and pepper as desired.

Recipe 5. Matcha Green Tea and Almond Biscotti

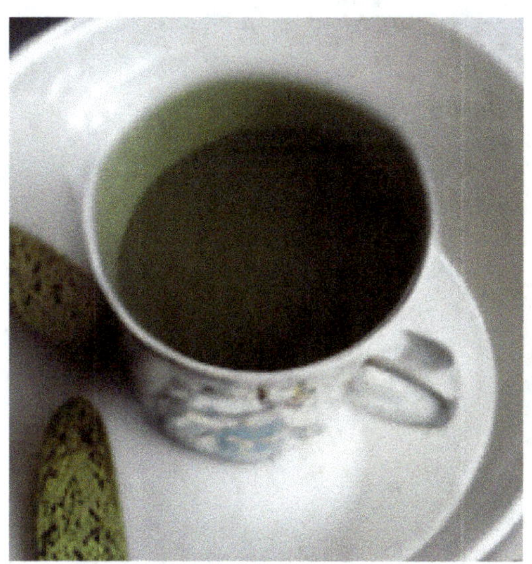

Ingredients:

- Almond flour
- Matcha green tea powder
- Almonds, chopped
- Maple syrup or agave nectar
- Almond extract
- Baking powder

Preparation:

1. Preheat the oven to 350°F (175°C).
2. In a bowl, combine almond flour, matcha green tea powder, chopped almonds, maple syrup or agave nectar, almond extract, and baking powder.
3. Form the dough into a log shape on a baking sheet.
4. Bake for 20-25 minutes or until golden.
5. Allow to cool, then slice into biscotti shapes.

Fruit-Centric Frozen Delights

Recipe 1. Mango Pineapple Coconut Popsicles

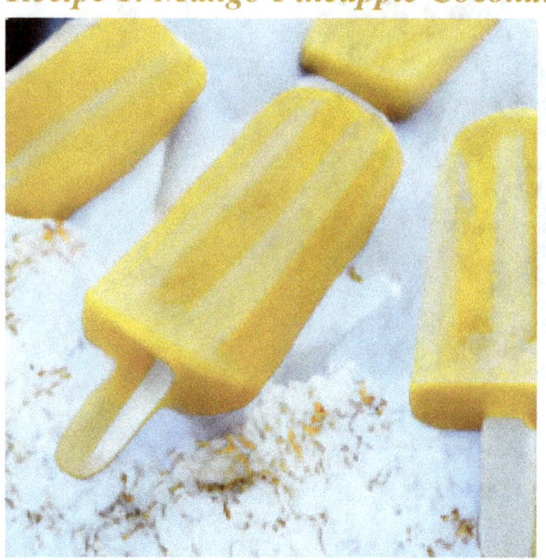

Ingredients:

- Ripe mango, peeled and diced
- Fresh pineapple, diced
- Coconut milk
- Agave nectar or honey
- Lime juice

Preparation:

1. In a blender, combine diced mango, fresh pineapple, coconut milk, agave nectar or honey, and lime juice.
2. Blend until smooth.
3. Pour the mixture into popsicle molds.
4. Place in the freezer for 4-6 hours, or until firm to the touch.
5. Unmold by briefly dipping the molds in warm water.

Recipe 2. Mixed Berry Yogurt Parfait Pops

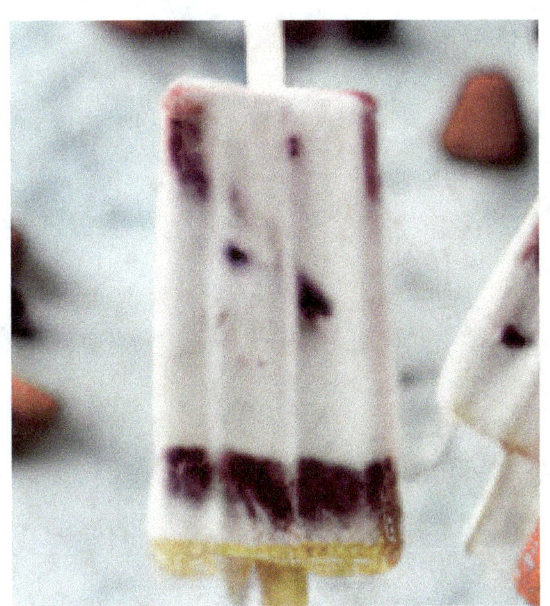

Ingredients:

- Mixed berries (strawberries, blueberries, raspberries)
- Greek yogurt or plant-based yogurt
- Honey or maple syrup
- Granola

Preparation:

1. In a bowl, mix mixed berries with honey or maple syrup.
2. In popsicle molds, layer the mixed berries with Greek yogurt or plant-based yogurt and granola.
3. Repeat the layers.
4. Insert popsicle sticks and freeze until solid.
5. Unmold by running under warm water.

Recipe 3. Watermelon Lime Sorbet

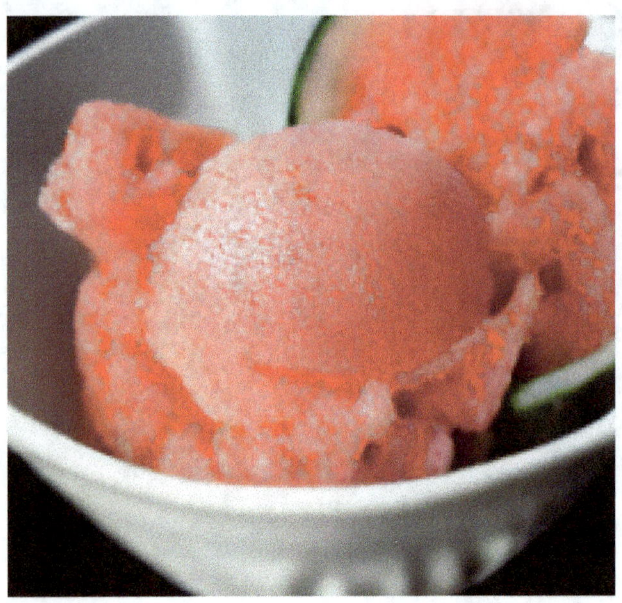

Ingredients:

- Mixed berries Fresh watermelon, seedless and cubed
- Lime zest and juice
- Mint leaves (optional)
- Agave nectar or honey (optional)

Preparation:

1. In a bowl, mix mixed berries with honey or maple syrup.
2. In popsicle molds, layer the mixed berries with Greek yogurt or plant-based yogurt and granola.
3. Repeat the layers.
4. Insert popsicle sticks and freeze until solid.
5. Unmold by running under warm water.

Recipe 4. Kiwi Coconut Chia Pops

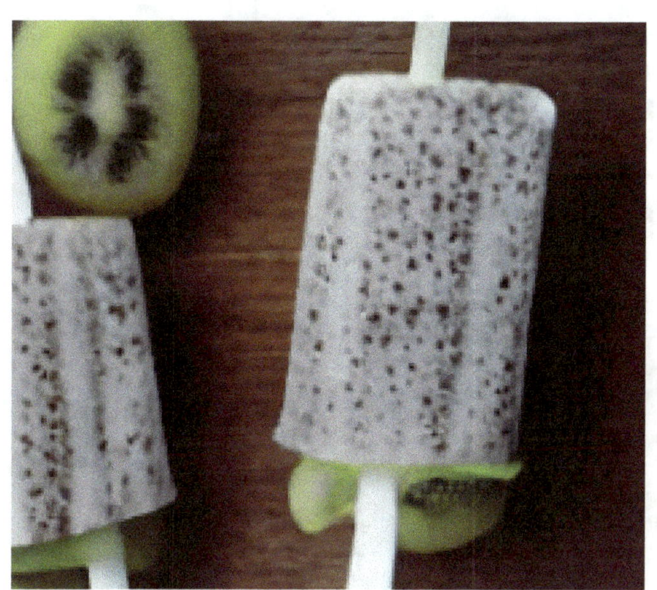

Ingredients:

- Kiwi, peeled and sliced
- Coconut water
- Chia seeds
- Agave nectar or honey

Preparation:

1. In a bowl, mix coconut water, chia seeds, and agave nectar or honey.
2. Let the chia mixture sit for at least 30 minutes to form a gel.
3. In popsicle molds, layer sliced kiwi with the chia mixture.
4. Insert popsicle sticks and freeze until solid.
5. Unmold by running under warm water.

Recipe 5. Passion Fruit and Mango Sorbet Swirl

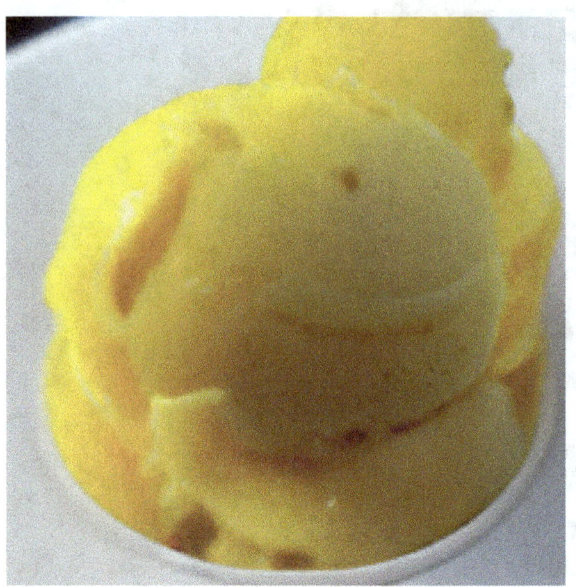

Ingredients:

- Passion fruit, pulp
- Ripe mango, peeled and diced
- Agave nectar or honey
- Lime juice

Preparation:

1. In a blender, puree passion fruit pulp with agave nectar or honey.
2. In a separate blender, puree diced mango with lime juice.
3. In popsicle molds, alternate layers of passion fruit and mango puree.
4. Skewer to achieve a swirled pattern.
5. Freeze until solid, then unmold.

Healthy Baking with Whole Plant-Based Ingredients

Recipe 1. Banana Walnut Oat Muffins

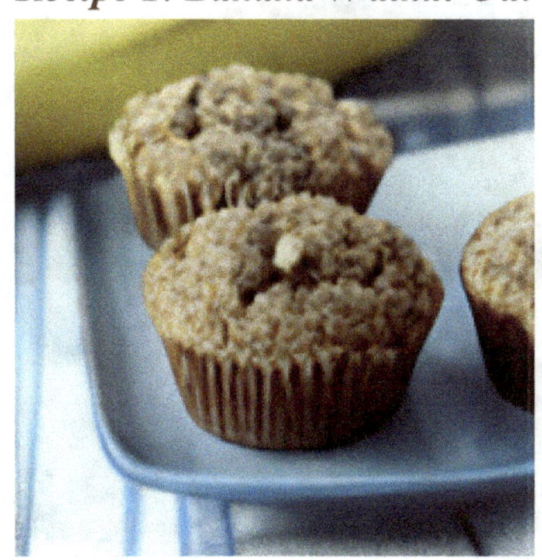

Ingredients:

- Ripe bananas, mashed
- Rolled oats
- Whole wheat flour
- Almond milk
- Walnuts, chopped
- Baking powder
- Cinnamon
- Vanilla extract

Preparation:

1. Preheat the oven to 350°F (175°C) and line a muffin tin with paper liners.
2. In a bowl, combine mashed bananas, rolled oats, whole wheat flour, almond milk, chopped walnuts, baking powder, cinnamon, and vanilla extract.
3. Mix until just combined.
4. Divide the batter into muffin cups and bake for 20-25 minutes or until a toothpick inserted comes out clean.

Recipe 2. Zucchini Carrot Breakfast Bread

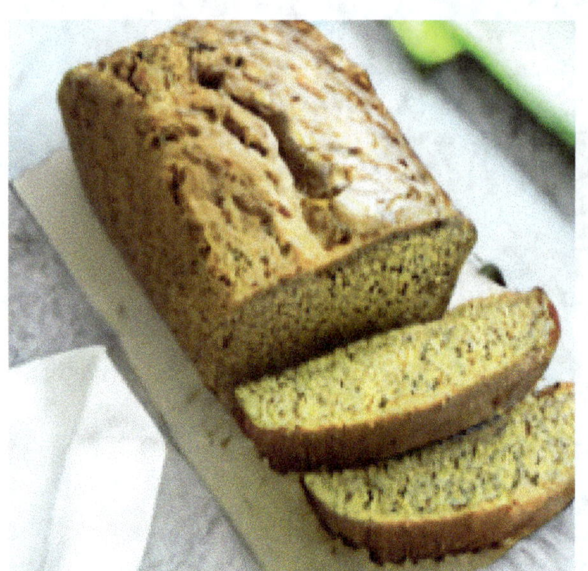

Ingredients:

- Shredded zucchini
- Shredded carrots
- Whole wheat flour
- Coconut sugar
- Almond butter
- Applesauce
- Baking soda
- Vanilla extract

Preparation:

1. Preheat the oven to 350°F (175°C) and grease a loaf pan.

2. In a bowl, mix shredded zucchini, shredded carrots, whole wheat flour, coconut sugar, almond butter, applesauce, baking soda, and vanilla extract.

3. Pour the batter into the loaf pan and bake for 45-50 minutes or until a toothpick comes out clean.

Recipe 3. Blueberry Chia Seed Muffins

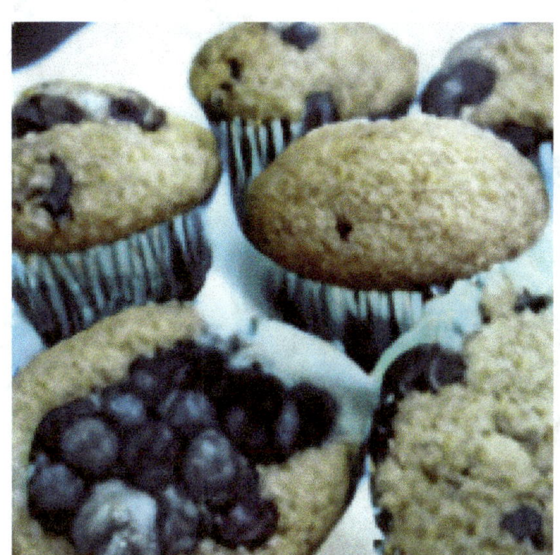

Ingredients:

- Blueberries, fresh or frozen
- Whole wheat flour
- Chia seeds
- Coconut oil
- Maple syrup or agave nectar
- Almond milk
- Baking powder
- Lemon zest

Preparation:

1. Preheat the oven to 375°F (190°C) and line a muffin tin with paper liners.
2. In a bowl, combine blueberries, whole wheat flour, chia seeds, coconut oil, maple syrup or agave nectar, almond milk, baking powder, and lemon zest.
3. Mix until well combined.
4. Fold in the blueberries.
5. Spoon the batter into muffin cups and bake for 20-25 minutes or until golden.

Recipe 4. Oatmeal Raisin Breakfast Cookies

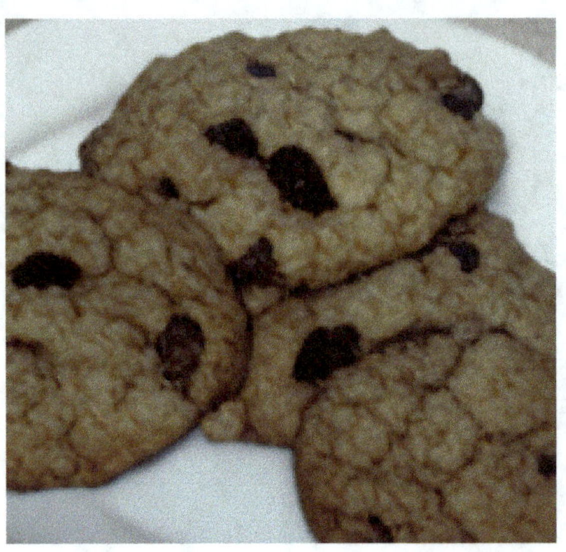

Ingredients:

- Rolled oats
- Raisins
- Mashed bananas
- Almond butter
- Flaxseeds
- Cinnamon
- Vanilla extract

Preparation:

1. Preheat the oven to 350°F (175°C) and line a baking sheet with parchment paper.
2. In a bowl, mix rolled oats, raisins, mashed bananas, almond butter, flaxseeds, cinnamon, and vanilla extract.
3. Scoop spoonfuls of the mixture onto the baking sheet.
4. Flatten each cookie with the back of a fork.
5. Bake for 15-18 minutes or until the edges are golden.

Recipe 5. Pumpkin Spice Quinoa Muffins

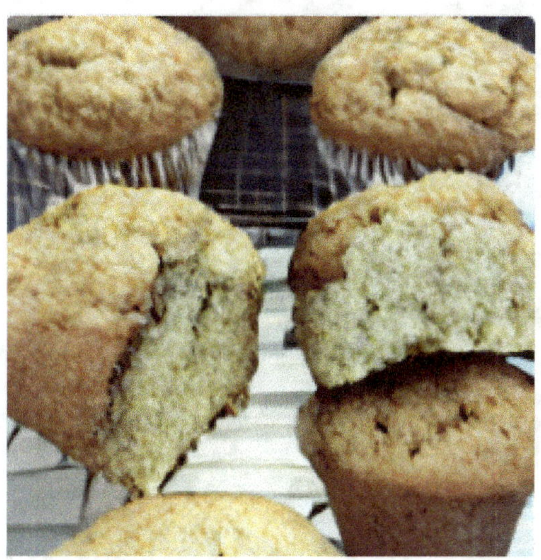

Ingredients:

- Cooked quinoa
- Pumpkin puree
- Whole wheat flour
- Coconut sugar
- Almond milk
- Pumpkin spice
- Baking powder
- Chopped nuts (optional)

Preparation:

1. Preheat the oven to 350°F (175°C) and line a muffin tin with paper liners.
2. In a bowl, combine cooked quinoa, pumpkin puree, whole wheat flour, coconut sugar, almond milk, pumpkin spice, baking powder, and chopped nuts if using.
3. Mix until just combined.
4. Divide the batter into muffin cups and bake for 20-25 minutes or until a toothpick comes out clean.

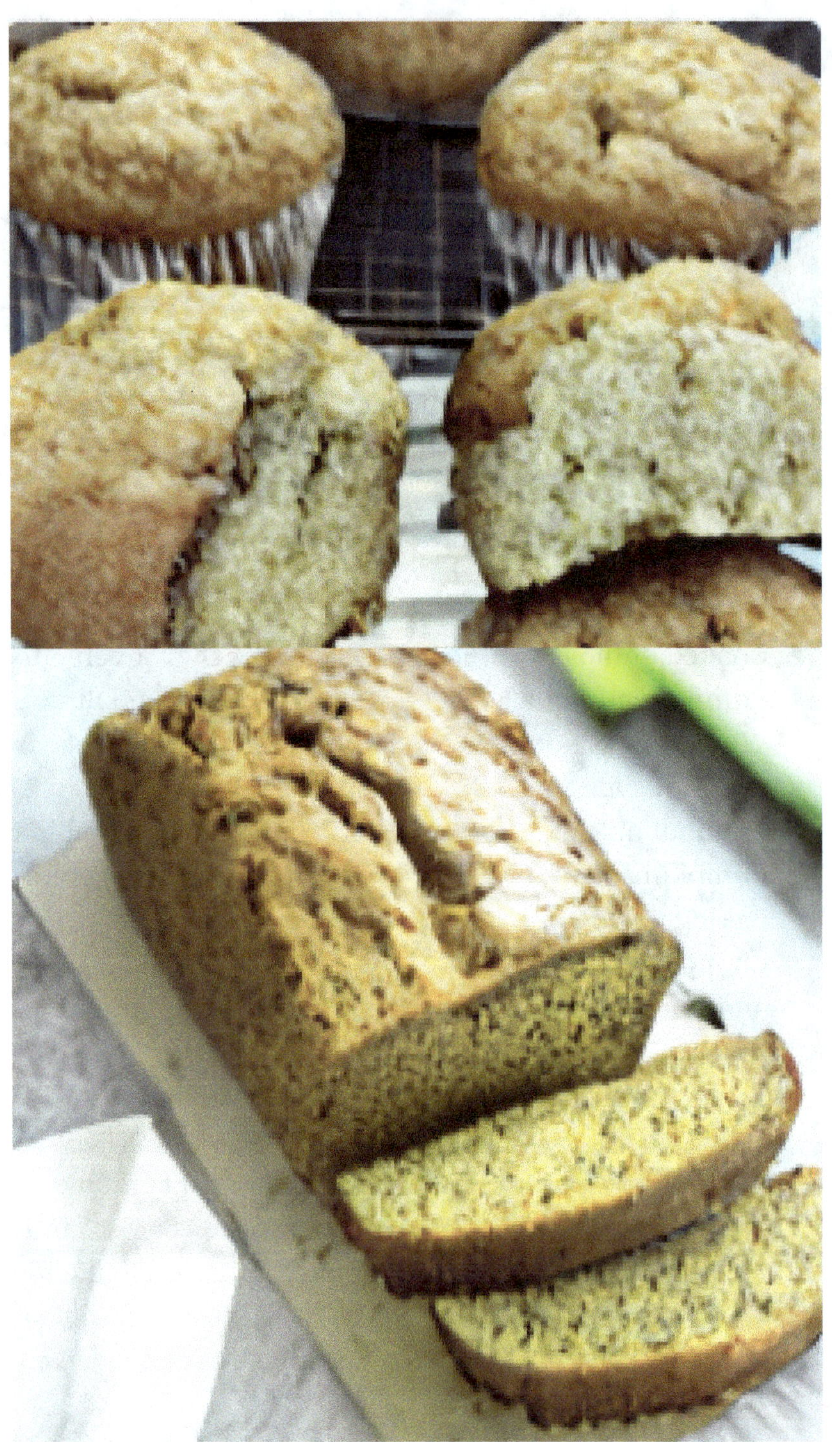

Chapter 8
Beverages to Boost Well-Being
Healing Herbal Teas and Infusions
Recipe 1. Chamomile Lavender Relaxation Tea

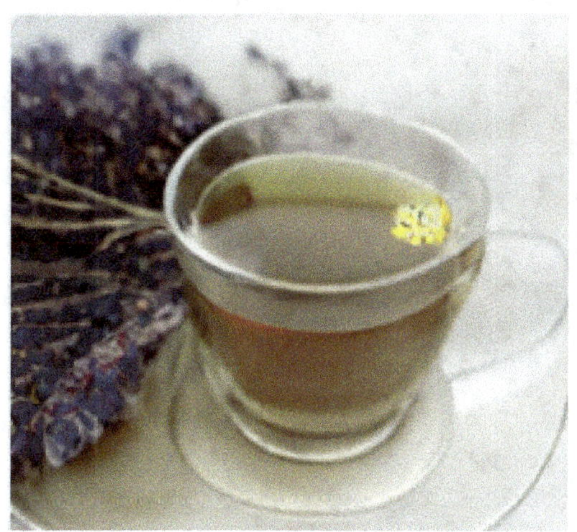

Ingredients:

- Chamomile flowers
- Lavender buds
- Peppermint leaves
- Honey or agave nectar (optional)

Preparation:

1. In a teapot, combine chamomile flowers, lavender buds, and peppermint leaves.
2. Infuse the herbs with hot water for 5-7 minutes.
3. Strain the tea into cups and sweeten with honey or agave nectar if desired.
4. Sip slowly and savor the calming blend.

Recipe 2. Ginger Turmeric Immunity Infusion

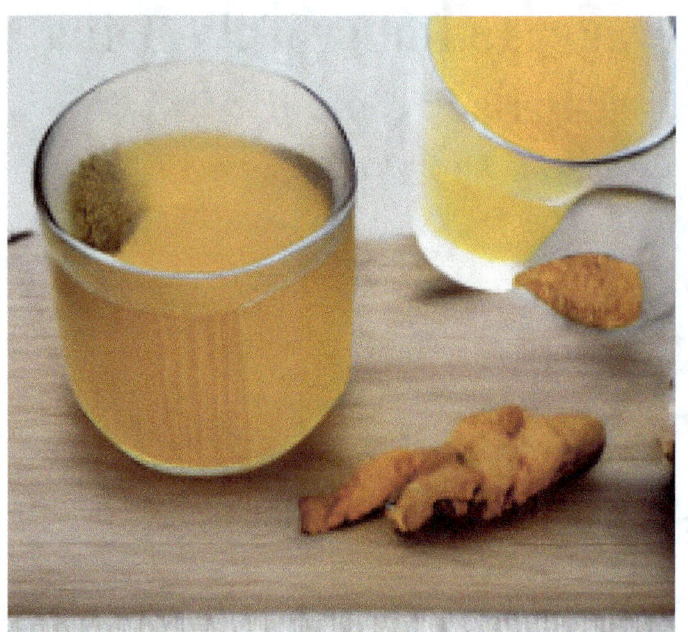

Ingredients:

- Fresh ginger, sliced
- Turmeric root, sliced
- Lemon slices
- Black pepper
- Honey or maple syrup (optional)

Preparation:

1. In a pot, combine fresh ginger, turmeric root, lemon slices, and a pinch of black pepper.
2. Add water and bring to a gentle simmer for 10-15 minutes.
3. Strain the infusion into mugs and sweeten with honey or maple syrup if desired.
4. Enjoy the immune-boosting goodness.

Recipe 3. Peppermint Eucalyptus Respiratory Tonic

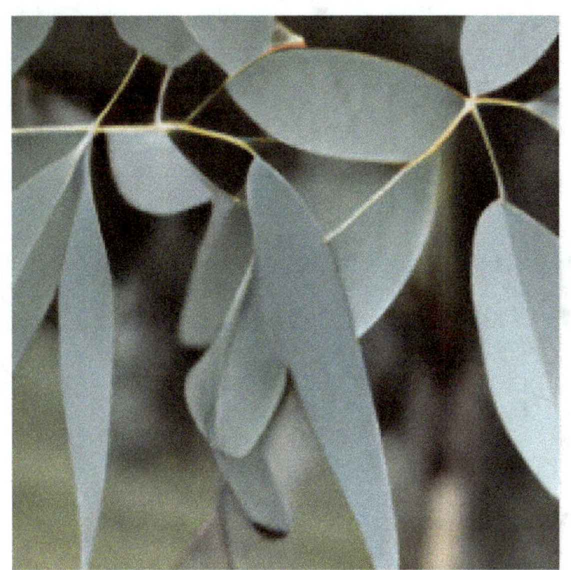

Ingredients:

- Peppermint leaves
- Eucalyptus leaves
- Lemon zest
- Honey or agave nectar (optional)

Preparation:

1. Steep peppermint leaves and eucalyptus leaves in hot water for 5-7 minutes.
2. Add lemon zest for a refreshing twist.
3. Strain into mugs and sweeten with honey or agave nectar if desired.
4. Inhale the aromatic steam for a soothing respiratory experience.

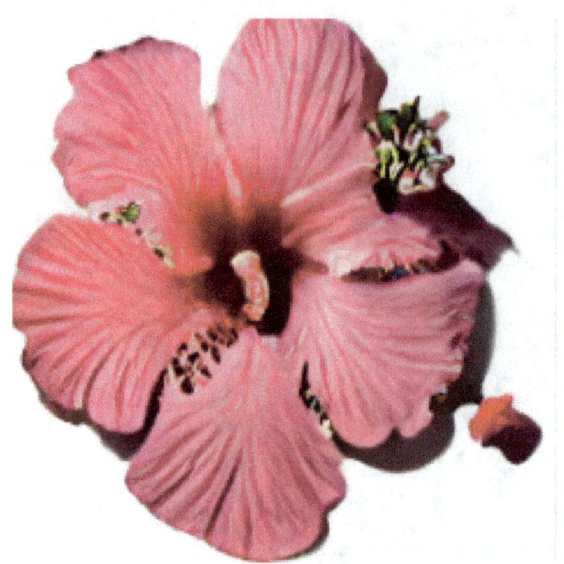

Ingredients:

- Dried hibiscus petals
- Rose petals
- Orange peel
- Cinnamon sticks
- Maple syrup or agave nectar (optional)

Preparation:

1. Brew a tea by combining dried hibiscus petals, rose petals, orange peel, and cinnamon sticks.
2. Allow the mixture to steep for 7-10 minutes.
3. Strain into cups and sweeten with maple syrup or agave nectar if desired.
4. Revel in the vibrant hues and floral aroma of this glowing elixir.

Recipe 5. Lemon Balm Lavender Bedtime Infusion

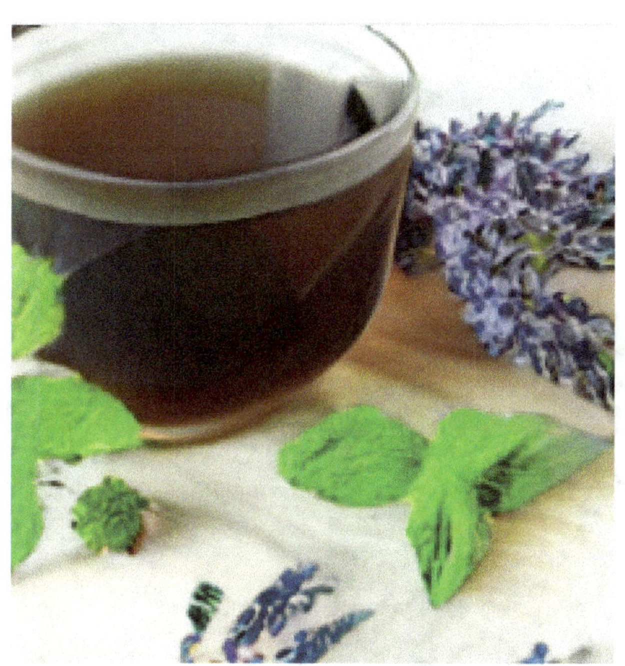

Ingredients:

- Lemon balm leaves
- Lavender buds
- Chamomile flowers
- Lemon slices
- Stevia or honey (optional)

Preparation:

1. Create a soothing infusion by steeping lemon balm leaves, lavender buds, and chamomile flowers in hot water.
2. Infuse with a hint of citrus brightness.
3. Strain into mugs and sweeten with stevia or honey if desired.
4. Wind down and enjoy this calming bedtime elixir.

Nutrient-Rich Smoothies for Every Occasion

Recipe 1. Green Goddess Detox Smoothie

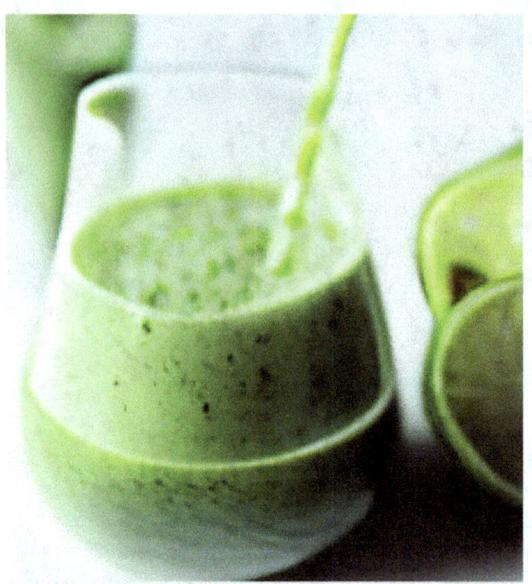

Ingredients:

- Spinach or kale leaves
- Cucumber, peeled and sliced
- Celery stalks
- Green apple, cored and chopped
- Fresh ginger, grated
- Lemon juice
- Coconut water or almond milk
- Ice cubes

Preparation:

1. Combine spinach or kale, cucumber, celery, green apple, grated ginger, and lemon juice in a blender.
2. Add coconut water or almond milk for liquid.
3. Blend until smooth.
4. Add ice cubes and blend again for a refreshing detoxifying smoothie.

Recipe 2. Berry Bliss Antioxidant Smoothie Bowl

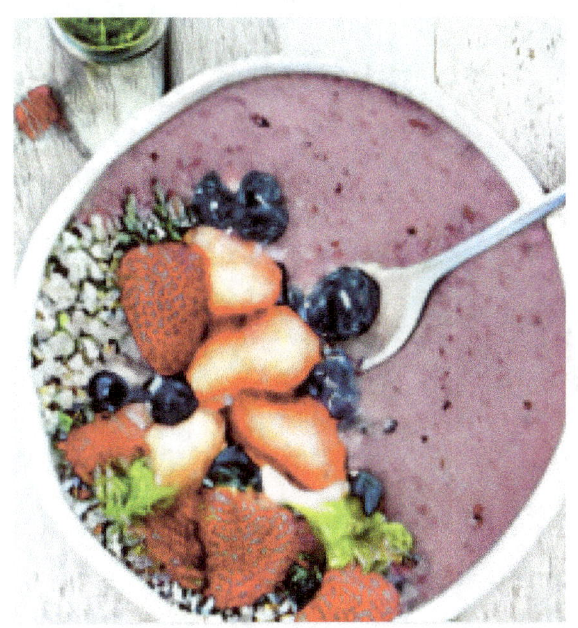

Ingredients:

- Mixed berries (strawberries, blueberries, raspberries)
- Banana, frozen
- Greek yogurt or plant-based yogurt
- Chia seeds
- Almond butter
- Almond milk
- Granola and fresh berries for topping

Preparation:

1. Blend mixed berries, frozen banana, Greek yogurt or plant-based yogurt, chia seeds, almond butter, and almond milk until smooth.
2. Pour into a bowl.
3. Top with granola and fresh berries for added crunch and antioxidant goodness.

Recipe 3. Tropical Paradise Energizing Smoothie

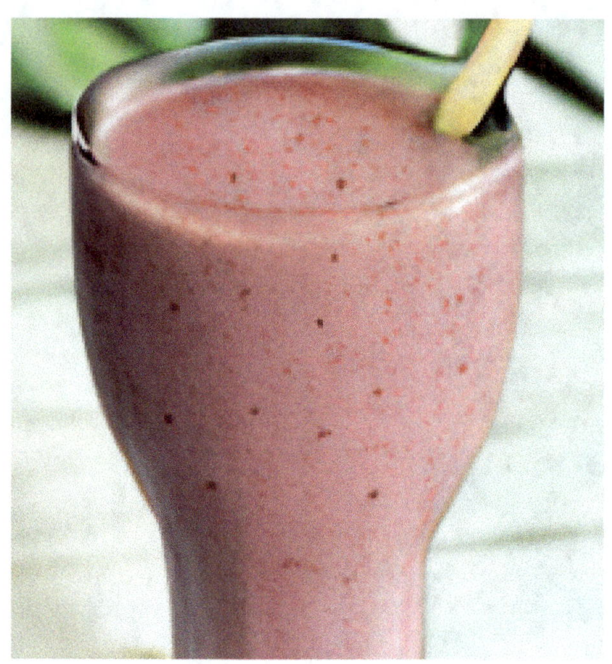

Ingredients:

- Pineapple chunks
- Mango, peeled and diced
- Banana
- Coconut water
- Fresh orange juice
- Turmeric powder
- Ice cubes

Preparation:

1. Blend pineapple chunks, diced mango, banana, coconut water, fresh orange juice, and a pinch of turmeric powder until creamy.
2. Add ice cubes and blend for a tropical and invigorating smoothie.

Recipe 4. Protein-Packed Peanut Butter Banana Smoothie

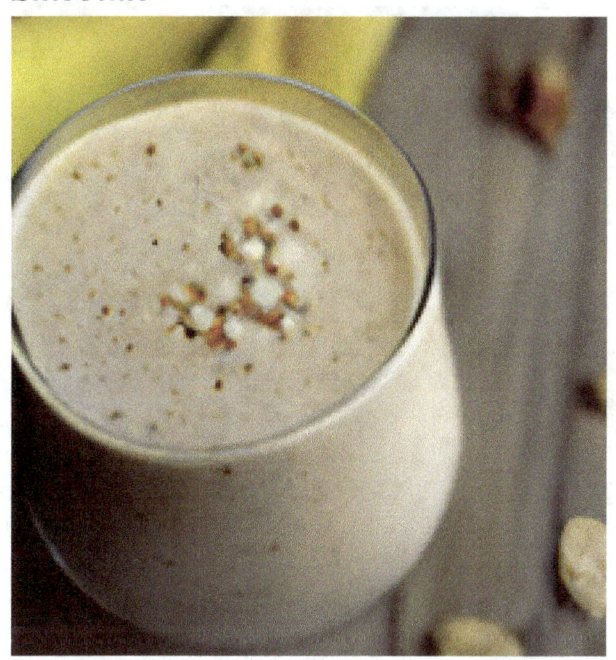

Ingredients:

- Ripe bananas
- Peanut butter
- Greek yogurt or plant-based yogurt
- Protein powder (vanilla or chocolate)
- Almond milk
- Ice cubes

Preparation:

1. Blend ripe bananas, peanut butter, Greek yogurt or plant-based yogurt, protein powder, and almond milk until well combined.
2. Add ice cubes and blend for a protein-packed and satisfying smoothie.

Recipe 5. Minty Watermelon Hydration Smoothie

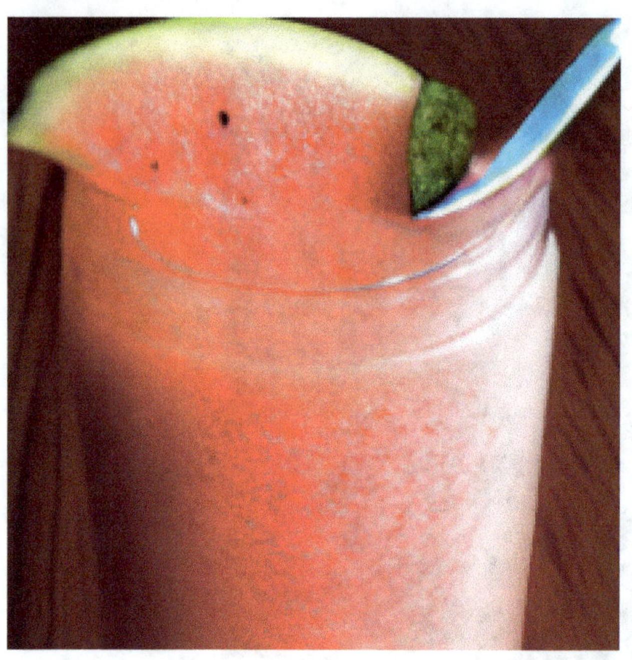

Ingredients:

- Watermelon, seedless and cubed
- Cucumber, peeled and sliced
- Mint leaves
- Lime juice
- Coconut water
- Ice cubes

Preparation:

1. Blend watermelon cubes, sliced cucumber, mint leaves, lime juice, and coconut water until smooth.
2. Add ice cubes and blend for a refreshing and hydrating smoothie.

Hydrating Infused Waters

Recipe 1. Citrus Mint Cooler

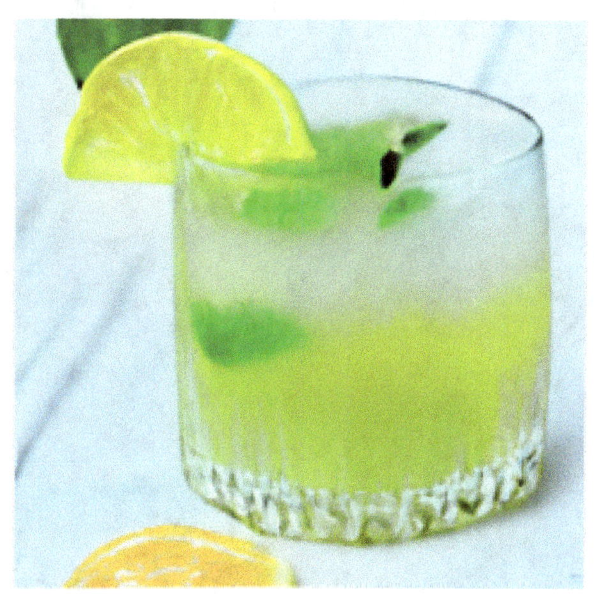

Ingredients:

- Lemon slices
- Lime slices
- Orange slices
- Fresh mint leaves
- Ice cubes
- Sparkling water

Preparation:

1. In a pitcher, combine lemon slices, lime slices, orange slices, and fresh mint leaves.
2. Add ice cubes for chill.
3. Top it off with sparkling water for a fizzy citrus-mint refreshment.
4. Stir gently and serve over ice.

Recipe 2. Cucumber Basil Infusion

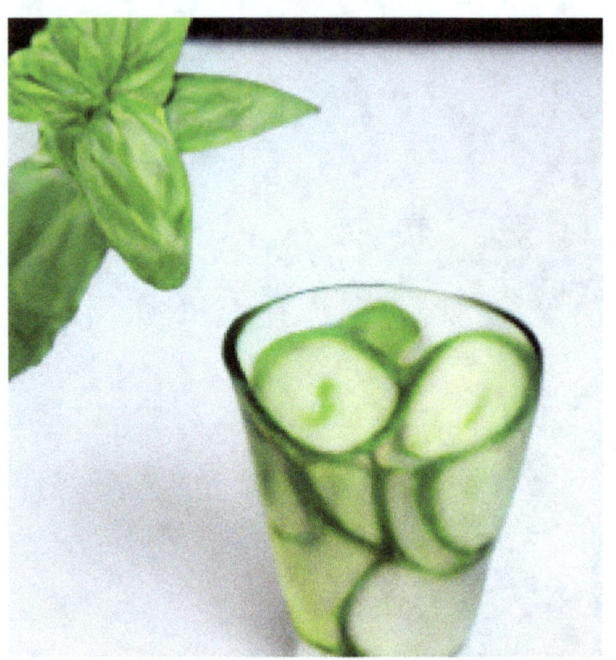

Ingredients:

- Cucumber, thinly sliced
- Fresh basil leaves
- Lemon slices
- Ice cubes
- Still or sparkling water

Preparation:

1. Place cucumber slices, fresh basil leaves, and lemon slices in a pitcher.
2. Add ice cubes for a crisp chill.
3. Fill the pitcher with still or sparkling water.
4. Allow the infusion to meld for at least an hour before serving over ice.

Recipe 3. Berry-Licious Hydration

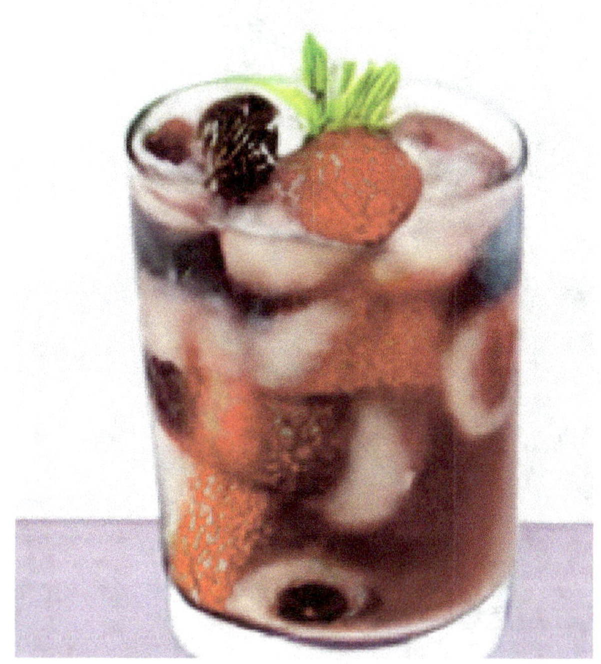

Ingredients:

- Mixed berries (strawberries, blueberries, raspberries)
- Lemon slices
- Fresh rosemary sprigs
- Ice cubes
- Still or sparkling water

Preparation:

1. Combine mixed berries, lemon slices, and fresh rosemary sprigs in a pitcher.
2. Add ice cubes for a refreshing chill.
3. Pour still or sparkling water over the ingredients.
4. Let the flavors meld for a few hours, then serve over ice.

Recipe 4. Pineapple Ginger Zing

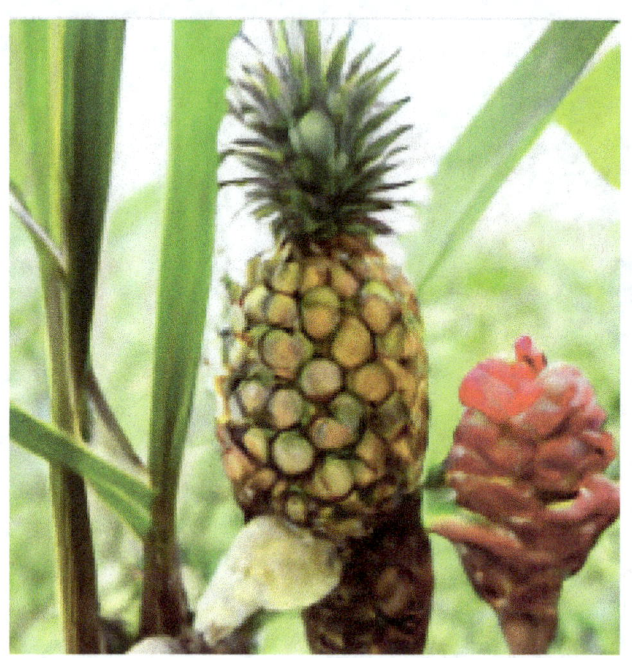

Ingredients:

- Pineapple chunks
- Fresh ginger, thinly sliced
- Mint leaves
- Ice cubes
- Coconut water

Preparation:

1. In a pitcher, mix pineapple chunks, thinly sliced fresh ginger, and mint leaves.
2. Add ice cubes for a cool kick.
3. Pour coconut water over the ingredients.
4. Allow the fusion to develop, then serve over ice for a tropical zing.

Recipe 5. Watermelon Basil Splash

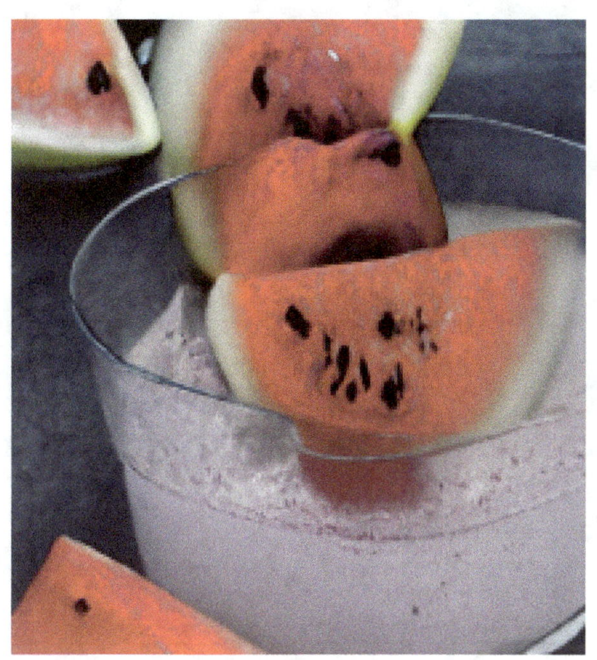

Ingredients:

- Watermelon cubes, seedless
- Fresh basil leaves
- Lime slices
- Ice cubes
- Still or sparkling water

Preparation:

1. Combine watermelon cubes, fresh basil leaves, and lime slices in a pitcher.
2. Add ice cubes for a cool splash.
3. Pour still or sparkling water over the ingredients.
4. Allow the infusion to meld, then serve over ice for a revitalizing splash.

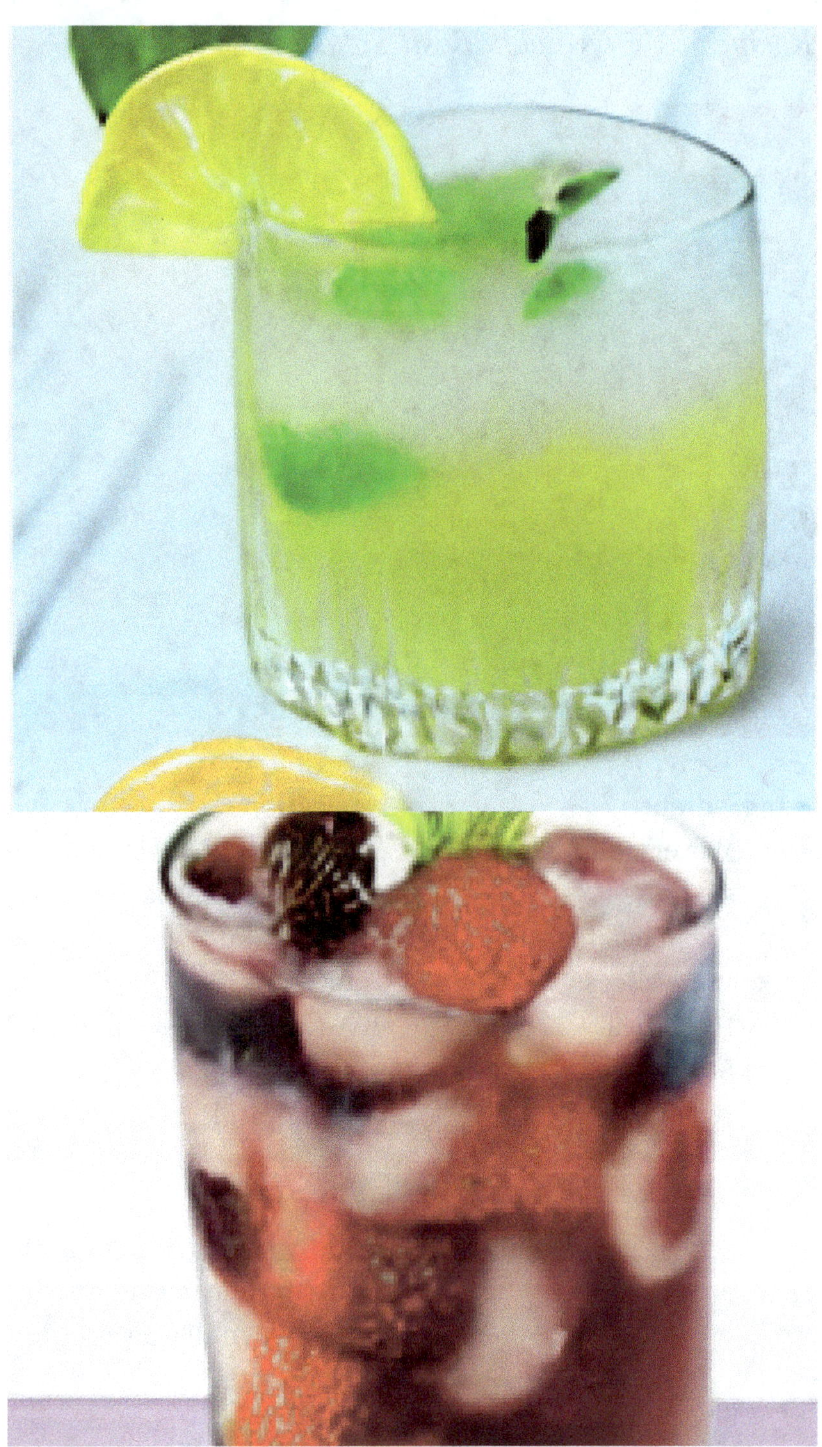

Chapter 9
Special Considerations
Plant-Based Eating during Cancer Treatment

Embarking on a plant-based journey during cancer treatment can be a transformative and empowering choice. In this chapter, we explore the nuanced considerations and thoughtful approaches to plant-based eating tailored to those undergoing cancer treatment. From managing side effects to ensuring adequate nutrition, these insights provide a compassionate guide to nourishing the body, supporting recovery, and fostering well-being during this challenging time.

Understanding the Landscape:

Living with cancer involves navigating a complex terrain of treatments, emotions, and lifestyle adjustments. As you consider embracing plant-based eating during this period, it's crucial to approach it with sensitivity and a focus on holistic well-being.

Key Considerations:

1. Nutrient-Rich Variety:
- Emphasize a diverse range of plant-based foods to ensure a broad spectrum of nutrients.
- Include a variety of colorful fruits, vegetables, whole grains, legumes, nuts, and seeds.

2. Adequate Protein Intake:
   - Incorporate plant-based protein sources such as legumes, tofu, tempeh, quinoa, and nuts.
   - Aim for a balanced protein intake to support muscle maintenance and overall health.

3. Managing Digestive Concerns:
   - Opt for easily digestible plant foods, such as cooked vegetables, soups, and smoothies.
   - Experiment with smaller, more frequent meals to manage digestive discomfort.

4. Hydration Importance:
   - Prioritize hydration, as it plays a crucial role in managing side effects and supporting overall health.
   - Infuse water with slices of fruits or herbs for added flavor and appeal.

5. Mindful Eating Practices:
   - Practice mindful eating to enhance the enjoyment of meals and promote a positive relationship with food.
   - Create a calm and supportive eating environment to foster a sense of well-being.

6. Consult with Healthcare Professionals:
   - Engage in open communication with healthcare professionals, including oncologists, dietitians, and other specialists.
   - Seek guidance on personalized dietary recommendations based on individual health conditions and treatment plans.

Empowering Through Plant-Based Choices:

Plant-based eating during cancer treatment can be a powerful tool for nurturing the body and promoting overall health. By embracing a thoughtful and balanced approach, individuals can harness the potential benefits of plant-based nutrition to support their well-being on physical, emotional, and spiritual levels.

Recipes for Resilience:

Explore a selection of plant-based recipes tailored for those undergoing cancer treatment. These recipes focus on gentle flavors, easy digestion, and nutrient density to provide nourishment during this challenging time.

1. Comforting Lentil Soup
   - Packed with protein and easily digestible, this warming soup offers comfort and nutrition.

2. Berry Banana Smoothie Bowl
   - A nutrient-rich and easy-to-enjoy smoothie bowl with a medley of berries and banana for added antioxidants.

3. Mashed Sweet Potatoes with Herbs
   - A soft and flavorful side dish rich in vitamins and minerals, providing both comfort and nutrition.

4. Ginger Turmeric Infused Water
   - A hydrating infusion with anti-inflammatory properties, offering a soothing option to stay hydrated.

5. Avocado and Chickpea Salad
  - A light and protein-packed salad featuring the creaminess of avocado and the nutrition of chickpeas.

Navigating a Path of Healing:

Plant-based eating during cancer treatment is a personal journey, and each individual's experience is unique. By embracing a mindful and compassionate approach, one can integrate plant-based choices to enhance the quality of nutrition, foster resilience, and contribute to a sense of empowerment on the path to healing. Always consult with healthcare professionals to tailor dietary choices to individual health needs and treatment plans.

Tailoring Recipes for Dietary Restrictions

Navigating dietary restrictions doesn't mean compromising on flavor or nutrition; it's an opportunity to explore creative culinary avenues. In this chapter, we delve into the art of tailoring recipes to accommodate various dietary restrictions, ensuring that everyone can enjoy delicious, nourishing meals regardless of their specific needs. From gluten-free alternatives to allergen-conscious options, these recipes cater to a diverse range of dietary preferences, fostering inclusivity and culinary delight.

Understanding Dietary Restrictions:

Dietary restrictions can stem from various factors, including allergies, intolerances, or specific health conditions. Whether it's gluten sensitivity, lactose intolerance, or other dietary considerations, tailoring recipes becomes a skillful art in addressing diverse needs without compromising on taste.

Key Strategies:

1. Gluten-Free Alternatives:
   * Explore gluten-free flours like almond flour, coconut flour, or a blend of rice and tapioca flour for baking.
   * Utilize naturally gluten-free grains such as quinoa, rice, and buckwheat as satisfying alternatives.

2. Dairy-Free Delights:
- Substitute dairy with plant-based alternatives like almond milk, coconut milk, or oat milk in recipes.
- Experiment with dairy-free butter, yogurt, and cheese options for diverse flavors.

3. Nut-Free Options:
- When faced with nut allergies, consider seeds like sunflower seeds, pumpkin seeds, or hemp seeds for added texture and nutrition.
- Seed butters, such as sunflower seed butter, can be excellent alternatives to traditional nut butters.

4. Plant-Powered Protein:
- For those following a vegetarian or vegan diet, incorporate plant-based protein sources like tofu, tempeh, legumes, and quinoa.
- Experiment with protein-rich vegetables like broccoli, spinach, and peas in various dishes.

5. Low-Carb Choices:
- Opt for low-carb alternatives like cauliflower rice, zucchini noodles, or spaghetti squash in place of traditional grains.
- Explore the richness of avocados and healthy fats for satisfying, low-carb options.

6. Allergen-Conscious Cooking:
- Be mindful of common allergens such as soy, eggs, and shellfish, and seek allergen-free alternatives when crafting recipes.

Recipes for All:

In this section, discover a selection of recipes tailored to accommodate various dietary restrictions. From a gluten-free banana bread to a dairy-free creamy pasta, these dishes celebrate inclusivity without compromising on taste or nutritional value.

1. Gluten-Free Banana Bread:
   - A moist and delightful banana bread made with a blend of gluten-free flours, ensuring a delicious treat for those avoiding gluten.

2. Dairy-Free Creamy Pasta:
   - A luscious pasta dish featuring a creamy, dairy-free sauce made from plant-based ingredients, offering a satisfying alternative to traditional cream-based dishes.

3. Nut-Free Energy Bites:
   - Energy-packed bites crafted with seeds and dried fruits, catering to those with nut allergies while providing a nutritious snack.

4. Protein-Packed Quinoa Salad:
   - A vibrant salad incorporating protein-rich quinoa, colorful vegetables, and a zesty dressing, ideal for those following plant-based diets.

5. Low-Carb Cauliflower Pizza:
   - A delicious pizza alternative with a crust made from cauliflower, allowing individuals to savor the flavors of pizza while keeping it low-carb.

Celebrating Diversity at the Table:

Tailoring recipes for dietary restrictions is a celebration of culinary diversity and inclusivity. By incorporating thoughtful substitutions and embracing a spectrum of ingredients, you create a dining experience that accommodates various needs without sacrificing the joy of flavorful, nourishing meals. Remember, open communication and awareness are key when catering to dietary restrictions, ensuring that everyone can indulge in the pleasure of good food.

Collaborating with Healthcare Professionals

Navigating the intersection of nutrition and health requires a collaborative effort between individuals, caregivers, and healthcare professionals. In this chapter, we explore the importance of working hand-in-hand with healthcare professionals to create personalized and health-conscious dietary plans. Whether managing chronic conditions, seeking weight management strategies, or addressing specific health concerns, this collaborative approach fosters informed decision-making and optimal well-being.

The Role of Healthcare Professionals:

Healthcare professionals, including doctors, dietitians, and nutritionists, play a pivotal role in guiding individuals toward dietary choices that align with their health goals and conditions. Collaborating with these experts ensures a holistic and evidence-based approach to nutrition.

Key Aspects of Collaboration:

1. Individualized Assessments:
- Healthcare professionals conduct thorough assessments, taking into account medical history, current health status, and dietary preferences.
- Tailored recommendations are based on individual needs, ensuring a personalized and effective approach.

2. Goal-Oriented Planning:
- Establishing health goals is a collaborative effort, with professionals guiding individuals in setting realistic and achievable objectives.
- Whether it's managing chronic conditions, achieving weight loss, or optimizing overall well-being, goals are tailored to each person's unique circumstances.

3. Nutritional Education:
- Healthcare professionals provide valuable nutritional education, empowering individuals to make informed choices about their diets.
- Understanding the nutritional components of food fosters a proactive approach to health and wellness.

4. Monitoring and Adjustments:
- Regular check-ins and monitoring help track progress and identify areas for adjustments in dietary plans.
- Flexibility is key, allowing healthcare professionals to adapt recommendations based on evolving health needs.

5. Lifestyle Integration:
- Collaborative efforts extend beyond dietary advice to encompass lifestyle factors such as physical activity, stress management, and sleep.
- A holistic approach addresses the interconnected aspects of well-being.

Navigating Specific Health Concerns:
This section explores collaborative approaches in managing specific health concerns through nutrition, offering insights into conditions like diabetes, cardiovascular health, and digestive disorders.

1. Managing Diabetes through Nutrition:
   * Collaborative strategies for optimizing blood sugar levels through balanced meal planning and mindful food choices.

2. Heart-Healthy Nutrition:
   * Insights into promoting cardiovascular health through dietary interventions, emphasizing heart-friendly choices and lifestyle modifications.

3. Supporting Digestive Wellness:
   * Collaborative approaches to address digestive disorders, focusing on dietary adjustments and nutritional support.

Empowering Health Through Collaboration:
A collaborative approach between individuals and healthcare professionals creates a powerful synergy, fostering informed decision-making and optimal health outcomes. By working together, individuals gain the knowledge and support needed to navigate their health journeys, making sustainable and positive changes to enhance their well-being. Remember, open communication and a shared commitment to health are the cornerstones of this collaborative partnership.

Navigating Specific Health Concerns:

This section explores collaborative approaches in managing specific health concerns through nutrition, offering insights into conditions like diabetes, cardiovascular health, and digestive disorders.

1. Managing Diabetes through Nutrition:
   - Collaborative strategies for optimizing blood sugar levels through balanced meal planning and mindful food choices.

2. Heart-Healthy Nutrition:
   - Insights into promoting cardiovascular health through dietary interventions, emphasizing heart-friendly choices and lifestyle modifications.

3. Supporting Digestive Wellness:
   - Collaborative approaches to address digestive disorders, focusing on dietary adjustments and nutritional support.

Empowering Health Through Collaboration:

A collaborative approach between individuals and healthcare professionals creates a powerful synergy, fostering informed decision-making and optimal health outcomes. By working together, individuals gain the knowledge and support needed to navigate their health journeys, making sustainable and positive changes to enhance their well-being. Remember, open communication and a shared commitment to health are the cornerstones of this collaborative partnership.

Conclusion

As we reach the culmination of this culinary odyssey, "Plant-Based Foods to Fuel the Cancer Fight," the journey has been more than a collection of recipes, it's been a transformative exploration of nourishment, resilience, and the boundless potential of plant-based eating.

In every chapter, we've delved into the intricate tapestry of nutrition, embracing the diversity of flavors, the richness of plant-powered ingredients, and the wisdom of tailored approaches to dietary needs. From understanding the profound connection between diet and cancer to crafting nutrient-rich smoothies for vitality, each segment has been a step towards fostering well-being and empowerment.

This book is not just a compilation of recipes; it's a guide, a compass steering you towards a path of vibrant health. It's an invitation to savor the goodness of plant-based foods that not only tantalize the taste buds but also contribute to the fight against cancer, inflammation, and a myriad of health challenges. It's about fostering a harmonious relationship with food, where each bite becomes a conscious choice towards wellness.

Through considerations for dietary restrictions, special circumstances during cancer treatment, and collaborative efforts with healthcare professionals, we've recognized the importance of inclusivity and informed decision-making.

As you embark on your culinary endeavors inspired by this book, remember that each recipe is a testament to the power of plant-based eating, a step towards fueling your body, mind, and spirit. Whether you're seeking comfort in a bowl of hearty soup, celebrating with a vibrant salad, or indulging in guilt-free snacking, every dish is an opportunity to nourish yourself with intention and purpose.

May these pages serve as a source of inspiration, a culinary companion in your quest for health, and a reminder that every choice you make in the kitchen is a small yet impactful step towards a healthier and more vibrant life. Let this book be your guide to embracing the nourishing power of plant-based foods, empowering you to fuel your own unique fight against the challenges life may present.

In the spirit of wellness, may your journey be filled with delicious discoveries, wholesome moments, and the resilience that comes from nurturing yourself with the incredible bounty that nature provides. Here's to savoring the flavors of life, one plant-based bite at a time, and to the vibrant health that awaits you on this nourishing path.

Thank you for being a part of this transformative journey. May your kitchen always be filled with the aroma of plant-powered possibilities, and may each meal be a celebration of the incredible fuel that plants provide for the journey towards radiant health.